HEALTHY EATING FOOD WHEEL

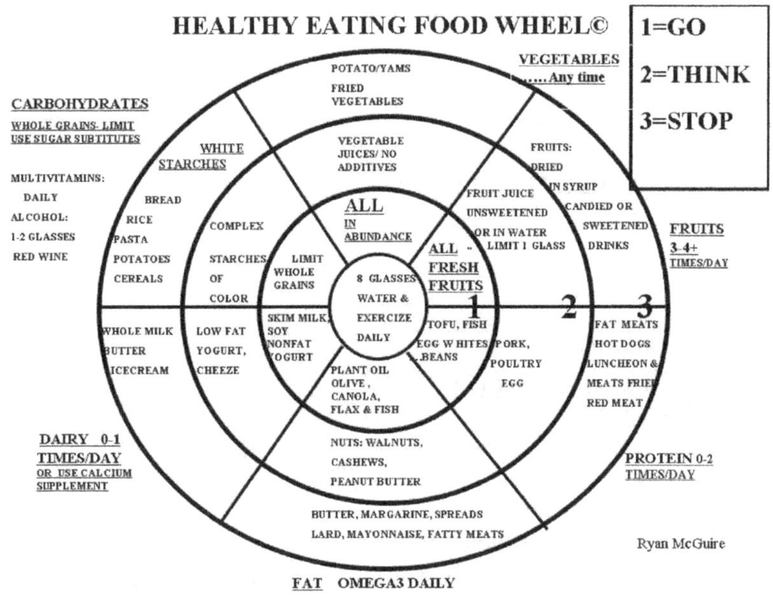

Ryan J. McGuire
MSN, FNP, CCE

ISBN 978-0-7414-3452-4

Published by:

INFINITY PUBLISHING

1094 New DeHaven Street, Suite 100
West Conshohocken, PA 19428-2713
Info@buybooksontheweb.com
www.buybooksontheweb.com
Toll-free (877) BUY BOOK
Local Phone (610) 941-9999
Fax (610) 941-9959

Printed in the United States of America

Published January 2012

Acknowledgments

I drafted this book during hurricane Katrina when I had occasion to review my studies in naturopathic nutrition in relation to the Food Wheel study at the VA Medical Center in New Orleans. I wish to thank the Food Wheel research team: Jamie Buth MD, Peter Holley NP, Rosemary Greenwood RD, Deborah Edwards NP, Gwendolyn Lemaire NP, and Denise Overby-Reyes NP for encouragement and stimulation. Thanks to Lorraine Landry, RSCJ and Cassandra McGuire for editing.

Notice

The Food Wheel is a guide to healthy eating and diet information. Recommendations are those of the author and are offered as guidelines within the context of the Food Wheel. Because the volume of data on many topics is extensive, they are not intended to be comprehensive or exhaustive. References are provided. The author, editors, and publisher do not warrant or guarantee the information contained, and do not assume and expressly disclaim any liability for errors, omissions, or consequences that may occur from use of this information.

CONTENTS

INTRODUCTION

Human obesity has its roots in the diet of Paleolithic man and its relationship to the diet of modern man. The diet of Paleolithic man represents thousands of years of evolution. The advent of modern mechanized agriculture took place about 150 years ago during the industrial revolution. Agricultural progress has caused diets to deviate from the diet of Paleolithic man. The introduction of foods not previously available such as refined grains, dairy, and new types of fats have become commonplace. After WWII, the increased use of processed foods contributed to the epidemic of obesity and chronic diseases that have become prevalent in our present industrialized and technologically advancing society.

The science of food (nutrition) is a new concept. Governments, the medical community, and business have intensified their study of nutrition for different reasons. The role of the government, to provide nutritional health standards for the American public, also has a role in promoting "agribusiness". Big business and big agriculture have increased research in order to market new and improved food products. Their marketing has had a significant influence on our view of appropriate food choices. The nutrition knowledge based on medical, government, business, and academic sources contain many diverse ideas about nutrition and diet. We, the public, are left to sort out these conflicting ideas of healthy eating and dieting.

This book proposes a healthy eating guide, The Food Wheel. The Food Wheel provides a pragmatic eating and buying guide based on current research and concepts. The Food Wheel also provides an explanation of macronutrients, micronutrients, digestion, glycemic load, glycemic index, energy density, satiation, and other underlying active principles of energy utilization. Each chapter is linked to the Food Wheel. Practical rules for shopping and dining are provided.

OBESITY: The Problem

The latest estimates in the United States indicate that 64% of adults are overweight and 31% are clinically obese. In 1976-1980, childhood obesity was only 5-6%. Now 10-15% of children are overweight. The International Obesity Task Force estimates that 1 billion people worldwide are overweight and 300 million are obese. Obesity is associated with higher mortality and increased risks of high blood pressure, heart disease, diabetes, gallbladder stones, osteoarthritis, and cancer. The prevalence of obesity has risen in the United States since WWII and markedly in the last 20 years. In developing countries, the rise in obesity is rapid. In countries that are beginning to adopt American fast and processed foods, obesity and its associated diseases are emerging. Increased caloric consumption and decreased activity in childhood have been implicated in adolescent and adult obesity.

Why are more children overweight? Very few children become overweight because of an underlying medical problem. Children are more likely to be overweight if their parents are obese. Genetic factors are thought to be less significant than the fact that families tend to share eating and activity habits. In other words, most children put on excess weight because their family lifestyles include an unhealthy diet and a lack of physical activity. It is easier now for children to become overweight because high calorie, energy dense foods are abundant, relatively cheap, and heavily promoted. Exercise, like walking, cycling to school, or playing sports is no longer a regular part of their daily routine. Children spend hours in front of a television or a computer. The National Diet and Nutrition Survey (2000) found that 40-69% of children over the age of six spend less than the recommended minimum of one hour a day doing moderate intensity physical activity.

A child's weight is classed as obese when their body weight is more than 25% fat in boys and 32% in girls. Children should never be placed on a weight-loss diet without medical advice. Unregulated dieting in teenage girls is thought to lead to the development of eating disorders. Children are encouraged to grow into their appropriate weight while eating healthier (provided there is a consensus as to what constitutes healthy eating) and increasing activity level.

The adult effects of learned childhood behaviors of over consumption and poor food choices can be seen by looking at adult indicators such as impaired fasting glucose (IFG) and impaired glucose tolerance (IGT) in the general population. IGF is a condition in which the fasting blood sugar level is elevated (100 to 125 milligrams per deciliter or mg/dL) after an overnight fast. Impaired fasting glucose tolerance (IGT) is a condition in which the blood sugar level is elevated (140 to 199 mg/dL) after a 2-hour oral glucose tolerance test. Under new guidelines published in the November 2005 issue of *Diabetes Care*, people with serial fasting blood sugars of >100 mg/dL and <126mg/dl are now considered to have prediabetes.

Data from U.S. adults aged 40-74 years who were tested for glucose levels from 1988 to 1994 was reviewed. The review showed that 33.8% had IFG and 15.4% had IGT. Therefore, 40.1% had prediabetes (IGT or IFG or both). If we used the 2000 U.S. population census of adults aged 40-74, we could estimate that greater than 41 million people have prediabetes. Long-term damage to the heart and circulatory system may already be occurring during prediabetes. This is important because consumption of high-energy dense foods promotes diabetes, high cholesterol, and obesity.

In the Diabetes Prevention Program, the development of diabetes was reduced 58% for persons who lost 5% to 7% of their body weight over 3 years using diet and exercising.

Prediabetic people treated with the diabetic drugs Metformin, Arcarbose, or a TZD, such as Avandia, have reduced their risk of developing diabetes. Such studies suggest that weight loss and increased physical activity prevent or delay onset of diabetes and related chronic diseases more than drugs alone. The problem is we are eating too much of the wrong foods.

Syndrome X is a metabolic syndrome that has become increasingly common in the United States. It is estimated that about 20–25 percent of US adults have it. According to the American Heart Association, Syndrome X is characterized by the following factors:

- Central obesity (excessive fat tissue in and around the abdomen). Men Greater than 40 inches.
  Women Greater than 35 inches.
- Atherogenic dyslipidemia (blood fat disorders of mainly high triglycerides and low HDL cholesterol that foster plaque buildups in artery walls). Fasting blood triglycerides greater than or equal to 150 mg/dL. Blood HDL cholesterol: Men less than 40 mg/dL Women less than 50 mg/dL
- Insulin resistance or glucose intolerance (the body cannot properly use insulin or blood sugar). Fasting glucose greater than or equal to 110 mg/dL.
- Prothrombotic state (e.g., high fibrinogen or plasminogen activator inhibitor in the blood)
- Raised blood pressure (130/85 mmHg or higher)
- Proinflammatory state (e.g., elevated high-sensitivity C-reactive protein in the blood)

The causes of Syndrome X are overweight/obesity, physical inactivity, and genetic factors. People are at increased risk of coronary heart disease, stroke, peripheral vascular disease, and type 2 diabetes.

There is another problem. The Department of Agriculture, one of the many federal agencies established to monitor and protect our health, is actually the agency responsible for promoting the products of American agribusiness. This can be conflicting when the USDA nutritional experts include representatives of the formidable meat, dairy, and sugar industries.

The USDA Food Guide Pyramid finalized in 1992, seen everywhere from the backs of cereal boxes to elementary school bulletin boards, has been proven a misleading dietary guide. The new 2006 guidelines is represented as an abstract pyramid that is web accessible only and linked to multiple pyramids according to individual calorie requirements. This is a distortion of what should be the single most important tool for improving the health of the nation. This contributes to misguided advice by health care professionals.

Meanwhile, the proliferation of a billion dollar popular diet industry has attempted to fill the information gap. Popular diets focus on a single aspect of diet such as low carbohydrate, low fat, or gimmick plans. Most of the published diet plans contain recipes instead of holistic nutrition information. The focus is on selling you their products. Unfortunately, popular diets have blurred the difference between nutrition science and nutrition pseudo-science.

The Food Wheel is based on all the current science and concepts embodied in revised food pyramids such as Mediterranean, Mayo, and Harvard diet plans. It addresses foundational information about the history of human nutrition from Paleolithic times to present. It explains all the food components and the function of digestion. It explores the basis for human metabolism and energy.

The Food Wheel is a pragmatic guide for the individual and the family to maintain healthy eating by making family changes of eating, shopping, and activity behavior.

PALEOLITHIC GENOME

Evolutionary biologists are aware that humans are genetically adapted to the dietary habits of their ancestors. The pre-agricultural times of collecting, hunting, and fishing started approximately 3 million years ago. One of the oldest bipedal humanoids, Homo erectus, is dated 1.8 million years ago. Profound changes in the human diet began in Mesopotamia with the introduction of agriculture and animal husbandry 10,000 years ago. The agro-industrial times began in England with the industrial revolution in the 19th century. That was only 150 years ago. After WWII, there was a technological revolution. Food changes accelerated with mass marketing of processed and packaged foods. We saw the explosion of a food consumer culture.

Let us put this in a time perspective of one year. If man appeared on earth on January 1, agriculture started on the second half of December of that same year, and the agro-industry started on December 31 late in the afternoon on the last day of that same year. These changes occurred too recently on an evolutionary timescale for the human genome to adjust.

Loren Cordain, PhD of Department of Health and Exercise Science Colorado State University has examined the dietary characteristics of humans living during Paleolithic times and historically studied hunter-gatherer societies. The mismatch between the contemporary human diet and our genetically determined physiology may be a significant contributor to obesity and the related diseases of civilization. We can compare the Paleolithic Diet and North American Diet by looking at proteins, carbohydrate, fat, and micronutrients.

In a Paleolithic diet, protein makes up about 25-30% of energy obtained almost exclusively from lean meats and fish.

The North American diet of today consists of 10-15% protein obtained from high fat meats, grains, dairy products and legumes. These present to the immune system protein fragments not known to pre-agriculture man. These new proteins are thought to play a role in autoimmune diseases such as Multiple Sclerosis, Rheumatoid Arthritis, Crohn's, Diabetes, and Celiac disease.

Paleolithic carbohydrates were obtained from fruits and vegetables, which have abundant micronutrients, high fiber, low amount of starches and sugars. They made up about 30-35% of the energy intake of Paleolithic humanoid. In the present North American diet, carbohydrates make up 50-60% of calories and are derived mainly from processed grains and refined starches. These new sources of carbohydrates achieve high blood sugar levels, which stresses the glucose-insulin system. Cereal grains are virtually indigestible by the human gastrointestinal tract without milling (grinding) and cooking. That is why the appearance of grinding stones in the fossil record generally heralds the inclusion of grains in the diet. Both the fossil record and ethnological studies of hunter-gatherers (the closest surrogates we have to Stone Age humans) indicate that humans rarely, if at all, ate cereal grains. The high phytate (a naturally occurring component of plant fiber) content of whole grain cereals can impair mineral metabolism. The high lectin content of whole grain cereals can allow intestinal antigens access to the peripheral circulation. Whole grain cereals are poor in vitamin C, vitamin B6, beta-carotene, and essential omega 3 fats. Human beings do not do very well when the total caloric intake of cereal grains approaches 70%. Hypogonadal dwarfism is found more often in populations consuming about 50% of total energy from unleavened whole grain breads. Ironically, whole grain cereals, which are promoted as more healthful than refined cereals because of their greater nutrient and fiber content, have a greater potential to disrupt mineral metabolism. However, low to moderate amounts of whole grains in the diet present little or no health problems to most people.

Fats comprised about 35-40% of Paleolithic energy and consisted mainly of monosaturated and polyunsaturated fats. Substantial amounts of omega 3 essential fatty acids (EFA) were consumed. The omega 6/omega 3 ratio ranged from 1:1 to 3:1. The main sources of fats were lean wild animals, fish, and nuts. Dairy products were not available until the advent of husbandry seventh and sixth millennia BC. Currently, the North American diet remains 35-40% fat but the ratio of omega 6 to omega 3 EFAs averages about 12:1. The fat types eaten today are saturated fat from fatty red meats, dairy products, and trans fatty acids from margarines and processed baked goods.

Micronutrients, such as vitamins, minerals, and antioxidants in the Paleolithic diet were about three times the present North American diet due to the increased consumption of fruits and vegetables. In addition, the North American sodium consumption (salt) is now about eight times that in the Paleolithic times.

The human dietary staple for more than 2 million years was lean game meat, seafood, fish, fowl, fresh fruits, and vegetables The human genome has changed relatively little in the past 40,000 years. It is not practical for contemporary men and women today to adopt and follow the exact dietary patterns of humans living during the Paleolithic times. It is imperative that we understand the significance of the Paleolithic Diet and its physiologic implications because, in essence, we are not biologically compatible with our present North American diet.

The Food Wheel reflects Paleolithic concerns by advising avoidance of refined carbohydrates, consumption of only moderate amount of whole grains, low fat dairy limited to once a day, and increased consumption of essential Omega-3 oil in fish, flaxseed, or canola. Limit sodium to 2000mg /day. Eat fresh fruits and vegetables anytime.

HISTORY OF NUTRITION

Early dieting: In the year 1087, King William the Conqueror began drinking alcohol in an attempt to lose weight in order to ride his horse. King William died that same year when his horse fell. Perhaps his drinking diet was successful because he did ride his horse again. Since then, there have been many diet plans and diet theories. It was not until recently that anyone had any understanding of the relationships between eating and obesity. People ate what they could grow, raise, catch, buy, barter, or steal. Three meals a day was unheard of. Remember, our bodies are essentially the same as those of our Paleolithic ancestors. Food eaten in excess of what is needed for energy, growth, or tissue repair was stored as fat for use later. Those whose bodies were most efficient at storing excess energy tended to live the longest and reproduce most successfully. Therefore, many years of natural selection pressures evolved humans into efficient utilizers of scarce food resources. The opportunity to store increasing amounts of energy as fat has been a common unpleasant fact only for the past few hundred years. The relationship of food to health was not well understood (Some would question whether it is well understood even today). People did not believe that it mattered what you ate. When there was enough food available for the average person to eat to excess, they got fat.

One of the first to write about diet in 1600 was Dr George Chayen, a Scotsman. In two essays, *An Essay of Health and Long life* and *English Malady*, he advocated a diet of milk.

Obesity began to be a more common complaint in the 1800s. That is why most early ideas about diet and dieting did not emerge previously. No one understood why some people got fat and others did not. No one knew what to do about it either. In 1811 Lord Byron, the poet, used vinegar to loose weight. In the early 1830s, an American minister by the name of Sylvester Graham preached that immorality was related to the sin of gluttony. His answer to good health was to follow a bland vegetarian diet. Graham advocated a life without coffee, tea, or other stimulants. He stressed a diet high in coarse-ground whole-wheat flour, which he baked into flat bread, referred to as graham crackers. This was very different from today's Nabisco gram crackers that contain 120 calories and 3 gram of fat in 2 crackers.

In England around 1850 William Banting, an undertaker, was the first person on record to follow a low carbohydrate diet and write about his experiences. Banting tried starvation, purgatives, diuretics, hot Turkish baths, and rigorous exercise. Some of the doctors that he consulted told him that obesity was simply incurable. Banting had occasion to consult Dr. William Harvey who recommended that Banting change his diet by cutting out most sugar and starch since foods containing those substances tend to create body fat. By following his low carbohydrate plan, Banting dropped fifty pounds. He wrote the world's first diet book in 1864 called *Letter on Corpulence Addressed to the Public*. **A low carbohydrate diet has been known for a century and a half**! Around the same time, Dr James Salisbury promoted a diet of hot water and meat patties, which become known as Salisbury steak.

The medical profession then had no idea how to treat obesity. They were sure everyone else was wrong just as they know the present popular diets are wrong. Before 1860, doctors in Paris had been finding successes treating Diabetes with the low carbohydrate approach. Our modern Diabetes experts, American Diabetes Association, and the US government are still blind to the plan. By the early 1890s, doctors who had previously thought obesity was incurable began to think of it as a disease caused by lack of thyroid hormone. Animal-based thyroid compounds started to be prescribed for weight loss in 1894. Since something could be given to treat obesity, people thought other things might also work. Common ingredients in these products were laxatives, purgatives, arsenic, strychnine, washing soda, and Epsom salts. Drug companies were born. Then in 1896, the first advertisements for products marketed exclusively for weight loss started to appear. Processed foods started to appear. In 1876, John Kellogg and his brother invented frosted corn flakes. In 1879, Monsanto Company invented the artificial sweetener Saccharin There was no turning back.

In the 1890s, chemist Wilbur Atwater and Russell Chittenden began to study foods and their energy values. They developed the idea of measuring the heat value of food by burning the components from each food group and measuring the amount of heat given off. The amount of heat that raised the temperature of one kilogram of water by one degree centigrade they called a calorie. The calorie was actually an estimate of the potential energy in food if it were burned. (We will discuss this relation to the laws of thermodynamics in detail later).

There have been countless diet plans. In the early years of the 1900s, American writer Upton Sinclair advocated fasting as a cure for both obesity and emaciation. A couple of years later, a spiritualist and magician named Harewood Carrington advocated eating only raw fruits and vegetables in his 1912 book, *The Natural Food of Man.* Horace Fletcher was the first to wear a white jacket to give him a look of authority. He apparently gleaned his diet ideas from a former British prime minister named William Gladstone who believed that prolonged chewing resulted in less overeating and improved health.

In 1919, a Los Angeles physician named Dr. Lulu Hunt Peters published her book entitled *Diet and Health, with a Key to the Calories*. This was the first book to advocate calorie counting as a method of weight reduction, and it had far-reaching effects. Dr. Peters promoted the "scientific principle" that calorie control equaled weight control. This was a gimmick to sell her book, which helped establish the erroneous idea that a measure of potential heat energy in food can adequately describe and predict metabolic energy utilization. (We will discuss this in detail in a later chapter). Dr. Peters can also be credited with starting the idea that being overweight is a sign of moral weakness. She sold two million books, making hers the first bestseller American diet book.

William H. Hay insisted that proteins, starches, and fruits had to be eaten separately to avoid acidosis. He urged one food category per meal, plus an enema every day. Gayelord Hauser's book, *Look Younger, Live Longer*, promoted his own line of special foods and supplements, stressing vitamin B-rich wonder foods, such as brewer's yeast, wheat germ, yogurt, powdered skim milk, and blackstrap molasses. Many of these ideas have resurfaced on TV or on the internet.

Before the mid-1800s, obesity was generally considered a bad luck situation for which there was no cure, short of near starvation. Meanwhile, developments such as the invention of Freon and improved agriculture production increased the availability of fresh food. Popular diet plans continued to promise a quick cure by focusing on one aspect of nutrition. In 1930, the Hollywood diet was introduced. It prescribed eating grapefruit, hard-boiled eggs, green vegetables, and Melba toast. This constituted about 600 calories. On a bright note, Wonder Bread, the first sliced bread, was introduced in 1930.

During the 1920s and 1930s there were many substances offered up as the answers to losing weight. Most of these included substances such as bladder wrack, kelp, and pokeberry. There remains today a plethora of herbs and chemicals advertised as miracle weight loss products.

Diets after WWII: The Great Depression stopped diet plan promotion. People had other worries. Then in the early 1940s came World War II, with food rationing and shortages. Ancel Keys received a government assignment at the start of World War II to design a lightweight but nutritious meal for the troops. A steady stream of diverse rations made their way through the developmental process. Two familiar rations introduced at that time were C and K rations. The K ration was created to cater to the needs of paratroopers, tank crews and other soldiers who depended on mobility for survival.

Both kinds of rations remained in service for decades, feeding troops in Korea and Vietnam. Research done in food science, preservation, and refrigeration were the beginnings of the revolution of food processing after WWII. For example, Greaves and Adair working at Cambridge University identified the freeze-drying process, which developed into the industrial process we know today.

It was not until the late 1940s and the early 1950s that weight loss programs began to reemerge. During this time, half of the medicines prescribed for obesity were speed (amphetamines).

In 1943, Marion White wrote a book called *Diet Without Despair* in which she advised her readers to use mineral oil in their foods. Mineral oil causes intestinal gas, bloating, and diarrhea.

Joan Nideth, in 1961, started meeting with friends to discuss weight loss. This was the beginning of Weight Watchers. In 1963, Tab was introduced as a sugar free drink.

In the 1970s, Dr. Robert Linn promoted his *The Last Chance Diet.* Fasting was broken several times a day by a small drink of the concoction that Linn had invented called Prolinn. Prolinn consisted of ground-up and crushed animal horns, hooves, hides, tendons, bones, and other slaughterhouse byproducts that were treated with artificial flavors, colors, and enzymes. Fifty-eight people were reported to have died from heart attacks while on the plan.

In the 1970s, Harvey and Marilyn Diamond promoted their book *Fit for Life* that proposed that our bodies have scientific needs categories of foods at certain hours of the day. Their plan included recommendations for eating only fruit before noon, and never eating protein at the same time as carbohydrates during the remaining hours of the day. The paperback edition sold over 3 million copies and claimed to be Americas #1 health and diet book.

In 1972, Dr Atkins introduced his low carbohydrate, high fat, and high protein diet. In 1978, Herman Tarnower published the Scarsdale high protein diet. The following year Nathan Pritikin published the *Pritikin Program for Diet &*

exercise which became popular with many cardiologists. In 1981, Judy Mazel publishes *The Beverly Hills Diet*, which proposed a fruit regimen. Then the Cambridge diet appeared. It consisted of low calorie and protein liquid drinks. Thirty people died of heart attacks due to nutritional deficiency. The popular Jenny Craig Company was formed in 1983. Dean Ornish reintroduced a low fat vegetarian diet Eat *More, Weigh Less* in 1993. Barry Sears published The *Zone*, which is a low carbohydrate diet and sparked a series of other low carbohydrate books such as *Sugar Busters*, *Protein Power*, and *The Carbohydrate Addict's Diet*. This represented a change in emphasis from low fat to low carbohydrate diets. In 2003, The South Beach Diet by Dr. Agatston struck a middle of the road approach. On the academic side several authors shed new light on dieting. Donald D Hensrud's book, *Mayo Clinic Healthy Weight for Everybody* (2005) redefined the food pyramid. WC Willett's book, *Eat, Drink, and be Healthy: The Harvard Medical School Guide to Healthy Eating* (2002) further redefined the food pyramid and helped introduce the concept of glycemic load. Miller Brand's book, *The Glucose Revolution: The Authoritative Guide to Glycemic Index* (1999) was foundational to the glycemic index and glycemic load. Before we explore these and other ideas related to the development of the Food Wheel, we will review the US government nutrition initiatives.

The US Government and Nutrition: The US Government was heavily involved in nutrition during WWII primarily to understand nutritional requirements for soldiers. After WWII the knowledge and technology was used for private enterprise. There was a proliferation of processed foods in bags, cans, and boxes. Fast foods replaced many of the natural foods such as fruits, vegetables, lean meats, and fish. The US Government was promoting nutrition standards. However, they were also promoting expansion agricultural and food processing industries.

The use of the scientific process to develop dietary guidance began at the U.S. Department of Agriculture

(USDA) with W.O. Atwater, the first director of the Office of Experiment Stations in USDA. In a Farmers' Bulletin published in 1902, Atwater emphasized the importance of variety, proportionality, and moderation in healthful eating the first USDA food guide, *Food for Young Children* by Caroline Hunt, a USDA nutritionist, appeared in 1916. This food guide, which specified five food groups, translated the emerging science of nutrition into recommendations for food intake.

Food guides emerged such as the "Basic Seven" (1946) and the "Basic Four" (1958). These guides focused on choosing enough of the kinds of foods to provide the nutrients needed for good health. The Basic 4 (milk, meat, vegetable and fruit, and bread and cereal) remained the centerpiece of nutrition education for the next two decades. Ancel Keys, the University of Minnesota public health scientist that developed K-rations, wrote with his wife in 1959 the cookbook, *Eat Well and Stay Well.* This was a message to eat less. After reviewing demographic nutrition data of data from seven of twenty-two countries, he noticed that countries with high saturated at consumption also had a high incidence of heart disease. He was the first to hypothesize a lipid connection to coronary heart disease (CHD). Years later, the American Heart Association officially incorporated his lipid theories into AHA dietary guidelines. Thus began the race for low fat diets and cholesterol lowering medicines.

The U.S. Senate Select Committee on Nutrition and Human Needs, popularly known as the McGovern Committee, set a new direction for dietary guidance in 1977 with the release of the *Dietary Goals for the United States*. This shifted the focus from obtaining adequate amounts of vitamins and minerals to avoiding excessive intakes of food components that had been linked to chronic diseases because there was a growing body of research relating over consumption of fat and sodium with the risk of heart disease and stroke. USDA did not adopt cautionary, eat less goals as the basis for food plans and guides because of opposition from senators and food industry. The USDA was already associated with big food industry lobby.

However, the Department of Health and Human Services (DHHS) asked the American Society for Clinical Nutrition (ASCN) to form a panel to study the relationships between dietary practices and health outcomes. The 1979 report was titled *Healthy People: The Surgeon General's Report on Health Promotion and Disease Prevention.* The report suggested that people reduce their consumption of excess calories, fat and cholesterol, salt, and sugar to lower disease rates.

In 1979, the USDA released a booklet the *Hassle-Free Guide to a Better Diet*. This guide added fats, sweets, and alcohol as a fifth food group to the Basic 4. The guide highlighted the need to moderate the use of fat, sugars, and alcohol and gave special attention to cutting calories and getting adequate dietary fiber.

All the previous eat less advisories were replaced in 1980 when DHHS and USDA published the first edition of *Nutrition and Your Health: Dietary Guidelines for Americans*. The guidelines called for a diet of a variety of foods to provide essential nutrients and more starch and fiber while maintaining recommended body weight and moderating dietary constituents of fat, saturated fat, cholesterol, sugars, sodium, and alcohol that might be risk factors in certain chronic diseases. These guidelines were directional rather than quantitative and were not acceptable to all nutrition scientists, health professionals, consumer groups, and food industry groups. One concern industry had was that the use of the term "avoid" would be interpreted to mean "eliminate" foods and result in an adverse economic impact.

A Federal Advisory Committee of nine nutrition scientists selected from outside the Federal Government was convened in 1983 to review and make recommendations to USDA and DHHS about this first edition of the *Dietary Guidelines*. In 1985, DHHS and USDA jointly issued a revised edition of the *Dietary Guidelines*. This second edition was nearly identical to the first. The changes were supposed to reflect advances in scientific knowledge of the associations between diet and a range of chronic diseases.

Now several agencies and congress get into the act. In 1987, a Conference Report of the House Committee on Appropriations indicated that USDA, in conjunction with DHHS, "shall re-establish a Dietary Guidelines Advisory Group on a periodic basis".

In 1989, USDA and DHHS established a second advisory committee that reviewed the 1985 Dietary Guidelines and made recommendations for revision in a report to the Secretaries of Agriculture and DHHS.

Marion Nestle managed the editorial production of the first and yet only *Surgeon General's Report on Nutrition and Health* published in 1988. No matter what the research indicated, the report could not recommend, "eat less meat" as a way to reduce intake of saturated fat, nor could it suggest restrictions on intake of any other category of food.

In 1989, National Research Council's report, *Diet and Health: Implications for Reducing Chronic Disease Risk* was a key resource used by the Dietary Guidelines Advisory Committee.

The 1988 Dietary Guidelines, conducted at the University of Wisconsin and The Pennsylvania State University under USDA sponsorship provided input from professionals and consumers.

In 1990, USDA and DHHS jointly released the third edition of the Dietary Guidelines. It contained, for the first time, suggested numerical limits for total fat and saturated fat intake.

Also, in 1990, The National Nutrition Monitoring and Related Research Act (7 U.S.C. 5341) was passed. This Act requires the Secretaries of Agriculture and Health and Human Services to publish jointly a report entitled Dietary Guidelines for Americans every 5 years.

In 1991 the Food Guide Pyramid (Fig 1), which was developed by USDA and supported by DHHS, was released. Secretary of agriculture blocked it. It took a year of negotiation with food industry and $855,000.00 to reach the compromise figure we now know! The Food Guide Pyramid has been widely used by nutrition educators in a variety of materials including posters, textbooks, school curricula, and computer software. It has also been used by industry on food labels The intent of the Food Guide Pyramid is to help consumers put the Dietary Guidelines into action but it was more a marketing statement than a representation of nutrition science. Essentially its message is all fats are bad and all carbohydrates are good.

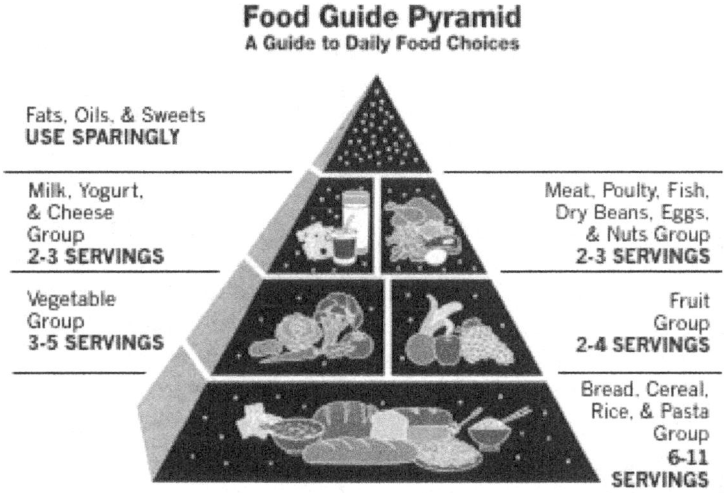

www.usda.gov

In 1994, USDA and DHHS appointed an 11-member Dietary Guidelines Advisory Committee to review the 1990 edition of the Dietary Guidelines and determine if, in consideration of current scientific knowledge, revisions were warranted. USDA and DHHS issued the 1980, 1985, and 1990 editions of the Dietary Guidelines voluntarily. The 1995 edition was the first report mandated by statute.

Although the titles of some of the Dietary Guidelines have changed, there have been few changes in the overall theme of the Dietary Guidelines over the past 25 years. All that has been accomplished is change in wording and presentation as you can see in the following table.

Dietary Guidelines for Americans 1980-1995

1980	1985
Eat a variety of foods Maintain ideal weight Avoid too much fat, saturated fat, and cholesterol Eat foods with adequate starch and fiber Avoid too much sugar Avoid too much sodium If you drink alcohol, do so in moderation	Eat a variety of foods Maintain desirable weight Avoid too much fat, saturated fat, and cholesterol Eat foods with adequate starch and fiber Avoid too much sugar Avoid too much sodium If you drink alcoholic beverages, do so in moderation
1990	**1995**
Eat a variety of foods Maintain healthy weight Choose a diet low in fat, saturated fat, and cholesterol Choose a diet with plenty of vegetables, fruits, and grain products Use sugars only in moderation Choose a diet moderate in salt and sodium If you drink alcoholic beverages, do so in moderation	Eat a variety of foods Balance the food you eat with activity Maintain or improve your weight Choose grain products, vegetables, and fruits Choose a diet low in fat, saturated fat, and cholesterol Choose a diet moderate in sugars and salt If you drink alcoholic beverages, do so in moderation

On Jan 2006 the below new USDA food guidelines were published: Compare those below to those above.

USDA Dietary Guidelines 2006

WEIGHT MANAGEMENT: To maintain body weight in a healthy range, balance calories from foods and beverages with calories expended. To prevent gradual weight gain over time, make small decreases in food and beverage calories and increase physical activity.

PHYSICAL ACTIVITY: Engage in regular physical activity and reduce sedentary activities to promote health, psychological well-being, and a healthy body weight. To reduce the risk of chronic disease in adulthood: Engage in at least 30 minutes of moderate- intensity physical activity, above usual activity, at work or home on most days of the week. For most people, greater health benefits can be obtained by engaging in physical activity of more vigorous intensity or longer duration. To help manage body weight and prevent gradual, unhealthy body weight gain in adulthood: Engage in approximately 60 minutes of moderate- to vigorous-intensity activity on most days of the week while not exceeding caloric intake requirements. To sustain weight loss in adulthood: Participate in at least 60 to 90 minutes of daily moderate-intensity physical activity while not exceeding caloric intake requirements. Some people may need to consult with a healthcare provider before participating in this level of activity. Achieve physical fitness by including cardiovascular conditioning, stretching exercises for flexibility, and resistance exercises or calisthenics for muscle strength and endurance.

ADEQUATE NUTRIENTS WITHIN CALORIE NEEDS: Consume a variety of nutrient-dense foods and beverages within and among the basic food groups while choosing foods that limit the intake of saturated and trans fats, cholesterol, added sugars, salt, and alcohol. Meet recommended intakes

CARBOHYDRATES: Choose fiber-rich fruits, vegetables, and whole grains often. Choose and prepare foods and beverages with little added sugars or caloric sweeteners, such as amounts suggested by the USDA Food Guide and the DASH Eating Plan. Reduce the incidence of dental caries by practicing good oral hygiene and consuming sugar- and starch-containing foods and beverages less frequently within energy needs by adopting a balanced eating pattern, such as the U.S. Department of Agriculture (USDA) Food Guide or the Dietary Approaches to Stop Hypertension (DASH) Eating Plan.

FOOD GROUPS TO ENCOURAGE: Consume a sufficient amount of fruits and vegetables while staying within energy needs. Two cups of fruit and 21/2 cups of vegetables per day are recommended for a reference 2,000-calorie intake, with higher or lower amounts depending on the calorie level. Choose a variety of fruits and vegetables each day. In particular, select from all five vegetable subgroups (dark green, orange, legumes, starchy vegetables, and other vegetables) several times a week. Consume 3 or more ounce-equivalents of whole-grain products per day, with the rest of the recommended grains coming from enriched or whole-grain products. In general, at least half the grains should come from whole grains. Consume 3 cups per day of fat-free or low-fat milk or equivalent milk products.

FOOD SAFETY: To avoid microbial food borne illness: Clean hands, food contact surfaces, and fruits and vegetables. Meat and poultry should not be washed or rinsed to avoid spreading bacteria to other foods. Separate raw, cooked, and ready-to-eat foods while shopping, preparing, or storing foods. Cook foods to a safe temperature to kill microorganisms. Chill (refrigerate) perishable food promptly and defrost foods properly. Avoid raw (unpasteurized) milk or any products made from unpasteurized milk, raw or partially cooked eggs or foods containing raw eggs, or raw or undercooked meat and poultry, unpasteurized juices, and raw sprouts.

FATS: Consume less than 10 percent of calories from saturated fatty acids and less than 300 mg/day of cholesterol, and keep trans fatty acid consumption as low as possible. Keep total fat intake between 20 to 35 percent of calories, with most fats coming from sources of polyunsaturated and monounsaturated fatty acids, such as fish, nuts, and vegetable oils. When selecting and preparing meat, poultry, dry beans, and milk or milk products, make choices that are lean, low-fat, or fat-free. Limit intake of fats and oils high in saturated and/or trans fatty acids, and choose products low in such fats and oils.

SODIUM AND POTASSIUM: Consume less than 2,300 mg (approximately 1 teaspoon of salt) of sodium per day. Choose and prepare foods with little salt. At the same time, consume potassium-rich foods, such as fruits and vegetables.

ALCOHOLIC BEVERAGES: Those who choose to drink alcoholic beverages should do so sensibly and in moderation -- defined as the consumption of up to one drink per day for women and up to two drinks per day for men. Some individuals, including those who cannot restrict their alcohol intake, women of childbearing age who may become pregnant, pregnant and lactating women, children and adolescents, individuals taking medications that can interact with alcohol, and those with specific medical conditions, should not consume alcoholic beverages. Individuals engaging in activities that require attention, skill, or coordination, such as driving or operating machinery, should avoid alcoholic beverages.

You can see that in 25 years there has been essentially no change. It is another chapter in the history of food politics where food industry giants lobby government departments to make sure their health advice supports industry. We have a nation of rising diabetes and obesity, and our own government will not tell people to eat less of anything. The message from the USDA has always been to eat more. Any ideas why this is the case?

According to federal regulations, the panel that writes the dietary guidelines must include nutrition experts who are leaders in pediatrics, obesity, cardiovascular disease, and public health. Selecting the panelists is no easy task, and is subject to intense lobbying from organizations such as the National Dairy Council, United Fresh Fruit and Vegetable Association, Soft Drink Association, American Meat Institute, National Cattlemen's Beef Association, and Wheat Foods Council. It resembles the situation at the FDA, where many of the people making the decisions on which drugs are approved are bankrolled by pharmaceutical companies. Majority of the people actually writing these dietary guidelines have financial ties to the very food industry groups that would be financially harmed by any advice telling Americans to eat less of anything. Can you spell C-O-R-R-U-P-T-I-O-N?

In contrast, scientists and physicians unencumbered by big industry have published volumes of research on various disease states and their relationship to the foods we eat. Why have popular diets become a billion dollar industry? If the USDA, the medical community, or drug companies had the answer to the increasing obesity and morbidity, these popular diets would have no market. Big government is more concerned with gross national product than with health. The importance is based on your consumer power not health status.

Marion Nestle's book, *Food Politics,* illuminates that nutritional problems of Americans can be traced to the food industry's imperative to encourage people to eat more in order to generate sales and increase income. (This is a must read book to get the flavor of the real politics of food).

Other organizations that purport to provide health standards are influenced by business interest. The American Heart Association (AHA) has received funding from cholesterol lowering drug manufacturers like Merck, Pfizer, Astra-Zeneca, and Bristol-Myers-Squibb. The American Heart Association has several hundred products bearing its famous 'heart-check' logo. The AHA earns millions of dollars from its "heart healthy" certification program. Some processed foods endorsed by the AHA makes one wonder what the heart healthy criteria really is. We will review their advice in a later section.

Examples of Foods Labeled as Heart Healthy

-Chocolate Moose Milk Chocolate Drinks;

-Malt-O-Meal Frosted Mini Spooners, Honey Graham Squares, and Honey Nut Toasty O's

-Kellogg's Frosted Mini-Wheats Big Bite

-General Mills Cheerios, Cocoa Puffs, Cookie Crisp, Corn Chex, and Count Chocula

-Healthy Choice Low Fat Ice Creams

-Kellogg's Nutri-Grain Cereal Bars

-Pop-Secret 94% Fat Free Butter Microwave Popcorn.

The American Dietetic Association (ADA) issues 'fact sheets' providing information on various nutrition and health topics underwritten by manufacturers such as Coca-Cola, Kellogg, Kraft Foods, Weight Watchers International, Campbell Soup, National Dairy Council, Nestle USA, General Mills, Monsanto, Nabisco, Procter and Gamble, Ross Products, Wyeth-Ayerst Labs, and Uncle Ben's.

The other ADA, American Diabetes Association, advises the consumption of carbohydrates and sugar for diabetic patients. The USDA food pyramid is its model along with portion control and exchange food lists. It advises that all foods are the same as defined by the calorie. Therefore, you can exchange one food for another as long as they are isocaloric. Patents are advised to reduce portions and to use the exchange lists to identify portion/calorie equivalent foods. The ADA states Glycemic Index does not have sufficient evidence based research and it has not addressed glycemic load or energy density (see glycemic index, glycemic load, and energy density in a later section). Hummm, ADA bases its advice on poorly supported evidence then states it needs a higher level of evidence to consider a change?

Other organizations are supposed to set standards for food related to disease states. The American Heart Association, and the U.S. Government's National Heart, Lung and Blood Institute were key proponents for acceptance of the anti-cholesterol high-carbohydrate hypothesis. The USDA's Food Guide Pyramid influenced millions of folks into believing that a high-carbohydrate grain-based diet was the epitome of healthy eating. The result of this advice is the increased level of obesity and type 2 diabetes.

Now, the USDA has paid 2.5 million dollars to produce this new abstract pyramid.

MyPyramid.gov
STEPS TO A HEALTHIER YOU

www.MyPyramid.gov

According to the USDA, it was designed to be simple. Details can be found only at the MyPyramid web site. What do the stripes stand for and how many servings of each food group are recommended each day? Millions of Americans without access to a computer or the internet will have trouble getting these facts. This dismantles and buries the flawed USDA pyramid. Perhaps, this is not a bad thing.

Essentially, the USDA has buried the old pyramid in order to avoid answering any of the mounting objections.

POPULAR DIETS AND OBESITY

A number of popular diets focus on carbohydrates and some on fats. Some demonize fats, and warn against eating any. Here is a how some popular diet plans treat carbohydrates and fats.

High carbohydrate/low fat diets such as Ornish, Pritikin, and Food for Life. Have told us for years we've been hearing that eating a healthy diet means cutting back on the total amount of fat and eating more complex carbohydrates. Thousands of low fat products line supermarket shelves. Gram for gram, fat has more than twice as many calories as either protein or carbohydrates. Therefore, it seems logical that choosing low-fat products would help with weight loss. Often the low-fat products on supermarket shelves are packed with sugar and highly processed carbohydrates to make up for the taste that is lost when fat is removed. These low-fat alternatives often have just as many calories as the full-fat versions. Another problem is that many people mistakenly think that because a food is low in fat they can eat as much of it as they want without gaining weight. As far as the body is concerned, eat too much calories (whether from fat, carbohydrates, or protein), and you will gain weight.

Aside from weight loss, the popularity of low-fat food has broader implications for health. Commercially prepared low-fat foods tend to be rich in highly processed carbohydrates, which cause big spikes in blood sugar. As described in the section on the glycemic index, over time this can increase the chances of developing heart disease and diabetes. For example, in a study of 80,000 nurses, Harvard researchers calculated that replacing a given number of calories from polyunsaturated fat with an equivalent number from easily digested carbohydrates increased the risk for heart disease by over 50 percent. Other studies have found that a low fat, high-carbohydrate diet can worsen blood cholesterol and triglycerides levels, which are, risk factors for heart disease.

Low carbohydrate/high protein diets such as The Zone, Atkins, South Beach, and other diets are in opposition to low fat approach. For more than two decades, Dr. Robert Atkins preached and sold the gospel of proteins are good and carbohydrates are evil. There is some evidence to back the idea that a high-protein, low-carbohydrate diet may help people lose weight. Whether a diet that includes bacon, steaks, butter, cheese, and other foods with plenty of saturated fat is good for overall health is another matter. In theory, a high-protein/low carbohydrate diet could help increase satiety (that feeling of fullness). Fewer carbohydrates also avoid fast and high rises and falls in blood sugar, which also keeps hunger at bay. Together, these could help you avoid overeating and make you satisfied with fewer calories. Reductions happen when people drastically change what they eat. Two year-long studies published in the New England Journal of Medicine suggest that the benefits of a low-carbohydrate diet may last for six months or a year. These studies compared high fat, high-protein, low-carbohydrate diets with low fat, moderate-protein, and high-carbohydrate diets. In both studies, the low-carbohydrate approach produced more weight loss at six months. However, by the end of a year weight loss was similar with both diets. Many of the high-protein foods that people choose while on this type of diet (red and processed meats, cheese, and full-fat dairy products, for example) are high in saturated fat and low in vitamins and minerals. This may increase the risk for heart disease and colon cancer. Diets very high in protein (especially animal protein, like red meat) may also increase the risk for osteoporosis in women because the body takes calcium from the bone to neutralize the acids that build up in the blood as a result of digesting large amounts of protein.

The low fat case summary: The folks promoting low fat diets are clearly in the mainstream, inasmuch as they are fully supported by the American Heart Association, the

AMA, and the USDA among other prominent health-related institutions. Their position also has the benefit of being eminently logical, and thus intuitively appealing. High levels of cholesterol and triglycerides are clearly associated with cardiovascular risk. Saturated fats and trans fatty acids increase the blood levels of bad lipids. Further, fatty foods are loaded with far more calories than the same amount of non-fatty foods, and thus lead to obesity, which is a major risk factor for cardiovascular disease. It makes sense that strictly limiting the amount of fat in the diet should help individuals control both their weight and their blood lipid levels. There are plenty of clinical studies demonstrating that this is the case. There is some evidence that patients following an extremely very low-fat diet can experience some degree of reversal of their coronary artery disease.

Low carbohydrate case summary: For 30 years, Government and health care promoted low fat diets and recruited the American food production industry to produce low fat versions of every foodstuff. Why, then, are Americans getting so fat? It is because carbohydrates cause obesity and stimulate hunger. When we eat carbohydrates especially the rapidly absorbed, simple carbohydrates like sugar, potatoes, pasta, white rice, and anything made from refined flour, (you know, the good stuff) we stimulate the secretion of insulin. Insulin causes glucose to be rapidly absorbed into the tissues for fuel consumption. Any extra glucose that is not immediately needed for fuel is converted to and stored as, ta da, Fat. Once the glucose levels drop, the insulin levels rapidly fall. Two to four hours after a high carbohydrate meal, we suddenly crave more carbohydrates. The cycle repeats. We eat carbohydrates, store fat, get hungry, and seek out yet more carbohydrates. While assiduously sticking to a low fat diet, we get fat, and as a result, our cholesterol levels go up. Thus, the scientific basis for the low carbohydrate diet seems at least as sound as that for the low fat diet. By avoiding carbohydrates, we avoid the spike in insulin levels and we are no longer fat storing animals. Our metabolism transforms so that we primarily use our fat stores for fuel instead of ingested glucose. The fat literally melts away.

The final facts on fats and carbohydrates:

1. Your body will utilize carbohydrates first as they are readily converted to glucose.
2. The conversion of carbohydrates or protein to fat is 10 times less efficient than just storing fat.
3. One hundred calories of carbohydrates (about 25gm) requires 23 calories to convert and store as fat.
4. One hundred calories of fat (about 11 gm) requires only 2.5 calories to be stored.
5. Extra carbohydrates consumed spares fat utilization.
6. Extra fat consumption promotes fat storage.
7. Only low carbohydrates and low fat eating plan promotes weight loss.
8. Extra energy consumed is energy conserved.

Popular Diet Plans, Fats, and Carbohydrates

Diet plan	**Fat**	**Carbs**
Ornish, Pritikin	Very low (10%)	Very high
AHA Step I& II, DASH,	Low (20%-30%)	High
Weight Watchers	Low (20%-30%)	High
Mediterranean, Zone	Moderate (30%-35%)	Moderate
South Beach	Moderate (30%-35%)	Moderate
Sugar Busters	High (45% or higher)	Low
Protein Power	High (45% or higher)	Low
Atkins	High (45% or higher)	Low
FOOD WHEEL	**High omega 3 Low animal fat**	**Low**

The Food Wheel is based on nutrition science, which turns the USDA pyramid upside down. The food wheel is a pragmatic tool that guides your food purchases because we know we will eat whatever we buy.

WHAT MAKES US FAT

Have you ever wondered why for so many weight gain seems inevitable? You can thank your Paleolithic ancestors that the human body is excessively efficient. Natural selection dictated that those not able to utilize energy efficiently died. It just does not take that much energy to maintain the human body at rest. With moderate activity, the human body burns only about 12 calories per pound of body weight per day. That means that if you weigh 167 pounds, your body uses only about:

167 X 12 = about 2,000 calories per day

All food labels assume a 2,000-calorie diet. You may not require 2,000 calories to do everything you need to stay alive. (You can calculate your caloric needs in the next section). A typical car in the United States gets between 15 and 30 miles per gallon of gasoline. A gallon of gas contains about 31,000 calories. If a human being could drink gasoline, a human being could run more than 300 miles per gallon. That level of efficiency is the main reason why it is so easy to gain weight. You burn only about 100 calories per mile when you are running. If you eat the McDonald's Big Xtra meal, it contains 710 calories in the sandwich, 540 calories in the French fries, and 310 calories in the drink for a total of 1,560 calories. That is 78% of a 2000-calorie diet, 86.6% of an 1800-calorie diet, and 130% of a 1200-calorie diet.

One method of estimating your level of obesity in relation to risk is BMI. BMI calculates obesity according to the relationship of weight and height. A BMI less than 20 is considered a low BMI for most people. A BMI of *20-25* is considered good. It may indicate a healthy weight for most people. A BMI of greater than *25* is considered to be high for most people. A BMI of 30 or greater is considered obese and has associated increased health risks. A BMI table follows.

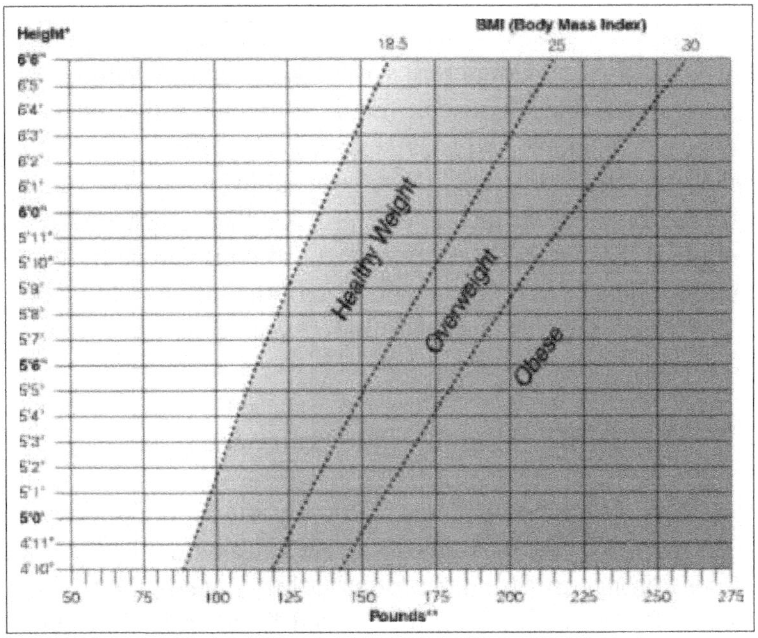

BMI =Weight [in pounds] x 704.5 / (Height [In inches]
Dietary guidelines 2000, www.fda.gov

If someone has a large muscle mass or is an amputee, the BMI will misstate the degree of obesity. Recent studies have shown that the amount of midline body fat may be a better predictor of the effects of obesity on health outcomes.

It only takes 3,500 excess calories to create 1 pound of new fat on your body. If you are taking in or losing just 500 extra calories per day, then you are gaining/losing a pound of fat per week (500 calories x 7 days = 3,500 calories). That is enough to raise the temperature of more than 10 gallons of water from the freezing point to the boiling point.

Dr. Jules Hirsch of Rockefeller University in New York proposed that people tend to end up at a weight that is specifically set for them in the brain called the set point.

Your metabolism increases when you gain weight and decreases when you lose weight. So, you tend to return to the same base weight.

There are five classes of drugs that are associated with weight gain. These can be prescribed alone or in combination and your primary care provider may not warn you:

1. Antidiabetes drugs
    a. Insulin
    b. Sulfonylureas: Glipizide, Glyburide, Amyrl
2. Antihypertension drugs
    a. Beta blockers: Propranolol
    b. Alpha-1 blockers : Terazosin
3. Antihistamines
    a. Cyproheptidine: used specifically to increase appetite
4. Psychiatric and neurological drugs
    a. Antipsychotic agents: Thioridazine, Olanzapine, Clozapine
    b. Mood stabilizers: Lithium
    c. Antidepressants: Amitriptyline, Nortriptyline, Imipramine, Martazapine, Paroxetine
    d. Antiepileptic drugs: Gabapentin, Valproate, Carbamzepine
5. Steroids
    a. Contraceptives
    b. Glucocorticoids

Food allergies have also been implicated in weight gain. The following foods are known to cause allergic reactions:

1. Milk and dairy products.
2. Wheat products.
3. Citrus fruits.

4. Eggs, corn, sugar, and chocolate.
5. Food coloring, additives, and preservatives.
6. Peas, peanuts.
7. Luncheon meats, sausage, ham, and bacon.
8. Caffeine in coffee, tea, and cola.
9. Vitamin, supplements, and OTC medications.

The theory of allergy related obesity is explained by brain response. After eating a food that is incompatible, there is an allergic reaction in which blood levels of serotonin decrease as part of the response. Consumption of energy dense carbohydrates and sugars cause a surge in insulin, which also increases tryptophan as a serotonin precursor. This produces a temporary feeling of well-being. The insulin causes a drop in blood glucose levels, which leads to subsequent seeking of carbohydrates and continued consumption of the offending foods. The offending foods are incorporated into the mix of energy dense foods we crave.

The determination of offending foods can be identified in two ways. The foods can be identified by a challenge diet where all possible offenders are removed then reintroduced one at a time. There is also a blood test called Alcat, which can identify food allergens. You can read about it at www.alcat.com. The test is expensive and requires someone trained in this area.

We are again reminded that foods or food additives may be incompatible with our physiology due to naturally accruing pharmacoactive chemicals, additives, and novel proteins. Food can be a powerful drug!

The introduction of novel proteins and other chemicals may contribute to our obesity problems. The Food Wheel returns us to natural fruits, vegetables, lean meats and fish. We avoid processed foods in bags, boxes, or cans. Today, food is just too easy to find. Remember, it was not so in as little as 150 years ago.

DIGESTION 101

Before we delve into specifics about food components, we will review how digestion works. Food placed in the mouth is chewed and lubricated by saliva secreted by three pairs of salivary glands. Small amounts of starch are digested by the amylase present in saliva. The resulting food is swallowed into the esophagus and is carried by peristalsis to the stomach. The stomach secretes 400-800 ml of gastric juice at each meal.

Three kinds of cells are found in the gastric glands: parietal cells, chief cells, and mucus secreting cells. Parietal cells secrete hydrochloric acid and intrinsic factor. Intrinsic factor is a protein that binds ingested vitamin B_{12} and enables it to be absorbed. The chief cells synthesize and secrete pepsinogen, which forms the proteolytic enzyme pepsin. Pepsin breaks long polypeptide chains into shorter lengths. Secretion by gastric glands is stimulated by the hormone gastrin with the arrival of food. Very little digestion occurs in the stomach except water, aspirin, and alcohol.

The contents of the stomach become liquefied and passes into the first 10-inch segment of the small intestine, the duodenum. Two ducts enter the duodenum. One drains the liver/gall bladder and the other drains the pancreas. The liver secretes bile, which is stored in the gall bladder until food enters the duodenum. A release of the hormone cholecystokinin (CCK) stimulates the gall bladder to contract and discharge its bile into the duodenum. Bile emulsifies globules of fat into tiny droplets that are more easily digested and absorbed. Bile pigments from old red blood cells impart the characteristic brown color of the feces.

Pancreatic fluid contains sodium bicarbonate, amylase, and lipase. The bicarbonate neutralizes the acidity of the fluid arriving from the stomach causing it to change to alkaline. Pancreatic amylase hydrolyzes starch into a mixture of maltose and glucose. Pancreatic lipase hydrolyzes ingested fats into a mixture of fatty acids and monoglycerides.

Intestinal blood drains into the liver. The liver has its own hepatic circulation system that serves as a gatekeeper between the intestines and the general circulation. The liver processes and detoxifies blood from the intestines before mixing with the general circulation. Monosaccharides are removed and converted into glucose. Excess amino acids are removed and broken down. The amino group is converted into urea. Glucose can enter the pathways of cellular respiration and be oxidized for energy or removed and converted into glycogen for storage. Many nonnutritive molecules, such as drugs and alcohol, are removed by the liver or detoxified. When the concentration of glucose in the blood drops, the liver releases more glucose by converting glycogen stores to glucose (glycogenolysis) and converting certain amino acids into glucose (gluconeogenesis).

The final digestion and absorption of sugars, reduced proteins, fatty acids, and monoglycerides occurs in the small fingerlike projections that carpet the inner surface of the small intestine, the villus. The surface of the epithelial cells of each villus is covered with microvilli (known as brush border). The total surface area of the intestine is almost 200 square meters, about the size of the singles area of a tennis court. The plasma membrane of the microvilli contain a number of enzymes that complete digestion by breaking down sugars proteins, and fats to their simplest components. Fructose simply diffuses into the villi. Sugars are absorbed by active transport. Fatty acids enter the cells of the villus and small droplets of fat are then discharged into the lymph vessels and transported to the liver.

The large intestine receives the residue water and indigestible cellulose. Bacteria flourish to such an extent that as much as 50% of the dry weight of the feces may consist of bacterial cells. Reabsorption of water is the chief function of the large intestine. The large amounts of water secreted into the stomach and small intestine by the various digestive glands must be reclaimed to avoid dehydration.

CALORIES

Calories apply to anything containing energy. Specifically, a calorie is the amount of energy, or heat, it takes to raise the temperature of 1 kilogram of water 1 degree Celsius. Most of us think of calories in relation to food, as in a can of soda, which has 200 calories. It turns out that the calories on a food package are actually kilocalories (1,000 calories = 1 kilocalorie). A can of soda containing 200 food calories contains 200,000 regular calories, or 200 kilocalories. This is also expressed as a measure of energy known as the joule. A (food) Calorie is equal to 1000 calories, or 4180 joules. The number of calories in a food is a measure of how much potential energy that food possesses. A gram of carbohydrates has 4 calories, a gram of protein has 4 calories, and a gram of fat has 9 calories. Foods are a compilation of these three building blocks. So, if you know how many carbohydrates, fats, and proteins are in any given food, you know how many calories, or how much energy, that food potentially contains if they were burned in a calorimeter.

If we look at the nutritional label on the back of a packet of maple-and-brown-sugar oatmeal, we find that it has 160 calories. This means that if we were to pour this oatmeal into a dish, set the oatmeal on fire and get it to burn the reaction would produce 160 Kcal, which is enough energy to raise the temperature of 160 Kilograms of water 1 degree Celsius. Our bodies "burn" the calories through metabolic processes, by which enzymes break the carbohydrates into glucose, the fats into glycerol and fatty acids, and the proteins into amino acids. These molecules are then transported through the bloodstream to the cells where they are either absorbed for immediate use or sent on to the final stage of metabolism in which they are reacted with oxygen to release energy in the cell mitochondria. The energy from fats, carbohydrates, and proteins are processed through different metabolic pathways. In the end, we can only say that extra energy consumed results in extra energy conserved.

Just how many calories do our cells need to function? The number is different for every person. You may notice on the nutritional labels of the foods you buy that the "percent daily values" are based on a 2,000-calorie diet. Height, weight, gender, age and activity level all affect your caloric needs. There are five main factors involved in calculating how many calories your body needs per day known as the total energy expenditure (TEE):

1. Amount of physical activity is 15-20% of energy.
2. Basal metabolic rate (BMR) and resting energy expenditure (REE) assumes a 12-24 hour fast. Basal energy expenditure (BEE) does not. The resting expenditure is 60-70%.
3. Thermic effect of food is about 10% but varies with the kind of food consumed.
4. Digestion and elimination processing is variable and depends on the kinds of food consumed.
5. Metabolic set point is variable by person.

Your metabolic rate (BMR/REE/BEE) is the amount of energy your body needs to function at rest. This accounts for about 60 to 70 percent of calories burned in a day and includes the energy required to keep the heart beating, the lungs breathing, the kidneys functioning and the body temperature stabilized. In general, men have a higher BMR than women. One method of calculating your basal metabolic rate is the Harris-Benedict formula:

Adult male: 66 + (6.3 x body weight in lbs.) + (12.9 x height in inches) - (6.8 x age in years)

Adult female: 655 + (4.3 x weight in lbs.) + (4.7 x height in inches) - (4.7 x age in years).

The second factor in the equation, physical activity, consumes the next highest number of calories. Your body burns an increased number of calories for about two hours after you have stopped exercising. The activity factors are multiplied by the BMR to adjust for activity level. Very light activity factor is 1.2-1.3 times BMR, light activity factor is 1.5-1.6 times BMR, moderate activity factor is 1.6-1.7 times BMR, and heavy activity factor is 1.9-2.1 times BMR. The energy in calories can also be roughly estimated by multiplying your weight in pounds Use 15 calories if you are active , 12 calories if you are inactive , and 13 calories if you are inactive and obese. For a 200 pound 60 year old male 71 inches tall the BMR by the Harris-Benedict formula for light activity calculates as 2366 calories. The rough estimate, 2400 calories, is close enough. That is a difference of calories in one slice of whole wheat bread.

The third factor is the energy needed to digest and eliminate foods. It is related to the amount of fiber and complex nature of foods. Natural foods, unrefined foods, raw foods, and foods high in fiber expend more energy to digest and eliminate.

The thermic effect of food is the amount of energy your body uses metabolically to process the food you eat. To estimate the number of calories you expend in this process, multiply the total number of calories you eat in a day by about 10 percent.

The set-point theory suggests that body weight is regulated at a predetermined level by a feedback control mechanism located in the hypothalamus. The controller integrates the information into a signal that modulates food intake or energy expenditure to correct any deviations in body weight from set point. When we increase our caloric intake, energy expenditure increases. When we decrease our caloric intake, our energy expenditure decreases. That is why after dieting, we gradually return to our previous weight.

Most diet controversy is about where calories come from. An excess of animal fat or refined carbohydrates can have serious health consequences. In the end, if we eat exactly the number of calories that we utilize do we remain even? The answer is a calorie is not a calorie.

When we are talking nutrition, it definitely matters where those calories originate. Different macronutrients of fat, carbohydrates, and proteins utilize different metabolic pathways.

LAWS OF THERMODYNAMICS

The misunderstanding that continues to be repeated in the expression "a calorie is a calorie" is a reference to the first law of thermodynamics. The first law is a conservation of energy law that states matter can neither be created nor destroyed. The first law states that in any transformation the total energy in the system can be accounted for by the heat added to the system, the work done by the system on its environment, and the change in energy content of all the components of the system. To understand the progress of a biophysical change it is necessary to understand the second law, which is a measure of disorder in all processes. The essence of the second law of thermodynamics is that it guarantees inefficiency in all metabolic processes, called entropy. There are different metabolic paths for fat, carbohydrates, and proteins. These are three different fuels metabolized differently. Therefore, energy balance is not to be expected in isocaloric diets that have equal calories but different food composition. It is important to understand that it is the second law that drives chemical reactions. The first law is a bookkeeping law and tells us that the total energy will be constant.

In weight loss diets, energy inefficient food is desirable. One component of inefficiency is the thermic effect of food. This is the energy used to metabolize food. We previously stated that this was about 10% of calories consumed. The thermic energy used to metabolize different macronutrients is approximately:

1. 2–3 % of calories for lipids.
2. 6–8 % of calories for carbohydrates.
3. 25–30% of calories for proteins.

As we decrease the grams of carbohydrates consumed the loss in calories to thermogenesis increases because the fat and protein we eat is used by the body for the manufacture of bile acids, hormones, enzymes, tissue, cell structure, and essential fatty acids. Macronutrients that are used to maintain body structure and function consume energy in the maintenance process of degradation, rebuilding and sparing a caloric source. The thermodynamic principles show that weight change on isocaloric diets is dependent on the metabolic path for each macronutrient. The kind of food consumed is just as important as the amount consumed.

The second law of thermodynamics guarantees variation of efficiency for different metabolic pathways. The popular dictum that a "calorie is a calorie" violates the second law of thermodynamics. A calorie is a measure of potential heat energy not metabolic energy.

Counting calories only holds as a general long-term rule of thumb where extra energy consumed results in extra energy conserved.

The two Food Wheel rules according to the Laws of Thermodynamics are:

1. **First law states, "If you eat too much you will get fat."**
2. **The second law states, "If you eat the wrong foods you will get fat."**
3. **The corollary states that, "a calorie is a calorie", "all fats are created equal", or "protein is protein" are incorrect.**

Remember, Dr. Lulu Hunt Peters' diet book in 1919 contributed to the popular calorie misconception. We will continue to use the term, calorie, while understanding that it is only an estimate of <u>potential heat energy</u> contained in food.

GLYCEMIC INDEX AND GLYCEMIC LOAD

The effects of different types of carbohydrates have generated the new concepts of glycemic index (GI) and glycemic load (GL). Dr. David Jenkins and a team of scientists at the University of Toronto system defined The Glycemic Index. The GI is a better method of classifying carbohydrates as it relies upon actual post-meal blood glucose response. The GI is a numerical system of measuring how fast a carbohydrate triggers a rise in serum glucose compared to a 50gm load of glucose standardized at a GI of 100. Some tables use bread standardized at 100. When you look at GI tables be sure you know if it is based on glucose or bread. GI bread standard is approximately 70% of GI glucose standard. A low GI food will cause a small/flat rise in blood glucose and a high GI food will cause a dramatic spike in blood glucose. A GI of 70 or more is high, a GI of 56 to 69 is medium, and a GI of 55 or less is low. High glycemic index foods have physiological consequences of hyperinsulinemia, insulin resistance, and increased pancreatic beta cell demand.

The disparity between the food volume and energy produced is not completely accounted for by glycemic index. Nutritionists at Harvard and in Australia have accounted for this by using the concept of glycemic load (GL). The GL assesses the impact of total carbohydrate and takes the GI into account. Glycemic load is the glycemic index divided by 100 multiplied by the available carbohydrate grams minus fiber grams. A GL of 20 or more is high, a GL of 11-19 is medium, and a GL of 10 or less is low. One GL unit is approximately equal to the effect of 1 gram of glucose.

This translates to a measure of the energy density of a given nutrient. For example, watermelon, known to be sweet, has a high GI of 72. A serving of 120gm has 6gm of available carbohydrates. However, the glycemic load is (72/100) x 6 = 4.32. The net effect on serum glucose is minimal.

GI/Gl curves are plotted by obtaining multiple blood samples from fasting volunteers who consume a prescribed amount of a food equal to 50gm of glucose.

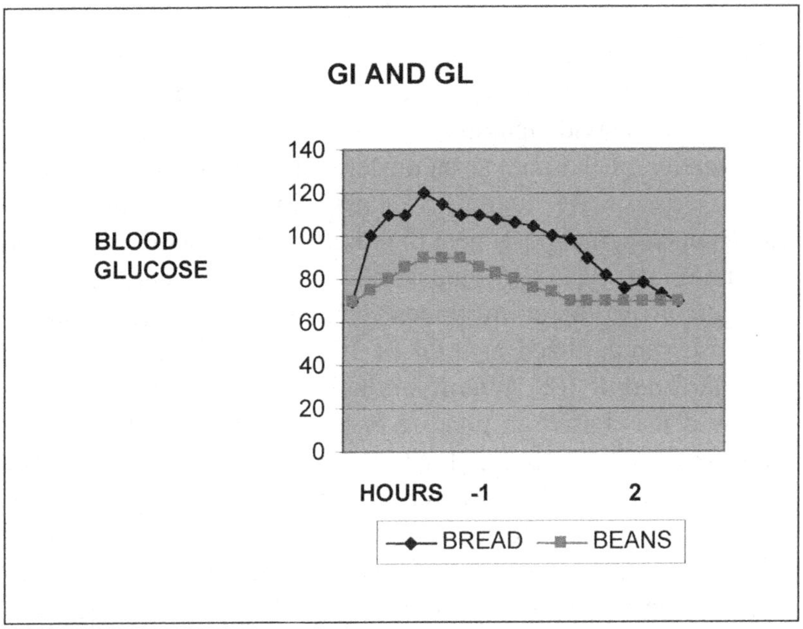

Glycemic load is the area under the curves, glycemic index is the rate of blood glucose increase. GL and GI are fundamental concepts of the food wheel.

Foods can have a combination of high or low GI and GL. High GI foods stress the system with a sudden influx of glucose. High GL foods require the body to manage excessive amounts of glucose. Therefore, there is short term and long-term effects of foods that have high GI/GL. Foods that have high GL but low GI process extra glucose if there is not over consumption. Foods with high GI but low GL are limited in their effects. Below is a table of some GI foods plotted against GL foods.

Glycemic index by glycemic Load

GI: LOW=1-55, MED=56-69, HI=>70
GL: LOW=1-10, MED=11-19, HI=>20

	LOW GI	MED GI	HI GI
LOW GL	All-brand Cereal 8,42 Apples 6,38 Carrots 3,47 Kidney beans 7, 28	Beets 5,64 Cantaloupe 4,65 Pineapple 7,59	Popcorn 8,72 Watermelon 4,72
MED GL	Bananas 12,52 Fettuccine 18,40 Orange Juice 12,50 Navy Beans 12,38	Wild rice 18,57 Life cereal 16,66 New Potatoes 12,57	Cheerios 15,74 Shredded wheat 15,75
HI GL	Linguine 23,52 Macaroni 23,47 Spaghetti 20,42	Sweet potatoes 27,61 White rice 23,64	Russet potatoes Baked 26,85 Cornflakes 21,81

You can use GI/Gl tables to count your daily GL points or use GI tables to calculate the total daily GL from the grams of carbohydrates consumed from each food. Foods with a GL less than 10 are listed in the following table.

<u>GL=GI/100 x grams carbohydrate minus grams fiber</u>

<u>Recommended Glycemic load for one day</u>

Weight less than 150 lbs .... Low GL 55 points
Weight 150-175 lbs .... GL 65 points
Weight >175 .... GL 80 points
High GL > 120 points .... Need to reduce carbohydrates

However, it is not necessary to count your daily GL points the Food Wheel guides you to eat foods with a GL of 10 or less. Fats and proteins do not have a significant GL.

Food list of most GL less than 10

Food:	GI	GL	Serving gm	Carbs gm
Apple, NS8 (Canada)	34	5.3	120	16
Apple, NS8 (USA)	40	6.2	120	16
Mean of six studies	38±2	5.5	120	15
Apple raw anytime				
Apple juice,	40	11.6	250	29
Limit juices				
Apple juice,	41	12.1	250	30
mean of three studies	40±1	11.2	250	28
Apricots, raw	57	5.2	120	9
Apricots, in syrup	64	12.0	120	19
Watch for canned fruits				
Apricots, dried30±7	8.0	60	27	
Apricots, dried	32	9.7	60	30
Most dried fruits have high GL				
Banana, ripe	51	12.9	120	25
Banana, under-ripe	30	6.3	120	21
Banana, over-ripe	48	12.1	120	25
Mean of 10 studies	52±4	12.4	120	24
Limit to one banana a day				
Cherries, raw,	22	2.7	120	12
Cranberry juice	16+			
Avoid excess juices				
Dates, dried	103±2	141.6	60	40
Avoid dried fruits				
Figs, dried,	61±6	15.7	60	26
Grapefruit, raw	25	2.7	120	11
Grapefruit juice	48	9.5	250	20
Grapes,	43	7.2	120	17
Mean of two studies	46±3	8.2	120	18
Grapes, black	59	10.5	120	18
Kiwi fruit, raw				
Mean of two studies	53±6	6.2	120	12
Mango				
Mean of three studies	51±5	8.5	120	17

Food:	GI	GL	Serving gm	Carbs gm
Oranges	48	5.4	120	11
Mean of six studies	42±3	4.6	120	11
Orange Juice	46±6	11.7	250	26
Avoid sweetened juices limit 1 glass/day				
Orange juice,	53±6	9.4	250	18
Orange juice,	57±6	15.1	250	26
Mean of three studies	52±3	12.1	250	23
Paw paw	56±6	4.7	120	8
Papaya	60	8.7	120	15
Mean of three studies	59±1	10.2	120	17
Peach, raw	28	3.7	120	13
Peach, raw	56	4.6	120	8
Mean of two studies	42±14	4.6	120	11
Peach, canned	30±4	3.4	120	11
Peach, canned	45±6	5.0	120	11
Mean of two studies	38±8	4.2	120	11
Peach, in syrup	52	9.2	120	18
Peach, syrup,	62±9	10.7	120	17
Pear, raw,	33	4.2	120	13
Pear, raw,	42	4.5	120	11
Mean of four studies	38±2	4.2	120	11
Pear halves, canned	43±15	5.4	120	13
Pear, canned	44	4.8	120	11
Pineapple, raw	66±7	6.3	120	10
Pineapple	51	8.0	120	16
Pineapple juice	46	15.4	250	34
Plum	53	5.7	120	11
Mean of two studies	39±15	4.8	120	12
Prunes, pitted	29±4	9.7	60	33
Prunes are ok				
Raisins	64±11	28.5	60	44
Avoid dried fruits				
Cantaloupe, raw	65±9	3.7	120	6
Strawberries, raw	40±7	1.3	120	3
Tomato juice, no sugar	38±4	3.5	250	9

Food:	**GI**	**GL**	**Serving gm**	**Carbs gm**
Watermelon, raw	72±13	4.3	120	6
Baked Beans, canned				
Mean of two studies	48±8	7.4	150	15
Beans, dried,	36	10.8	150	30
Beans, dried,	20	6.0	150	30
Mean of two studies	29±9	8.7	150	30
Black-eyed beans	50	15.2	150	30
Black-eyed beans highest GL				
Black-eyed beans	33±4	10.1	150	30
Mean of two studies	42±9	12.8	150	30
Butter beans, dried,	29±8	5.7	150	20
Butter beans	36±4	7.0	150	20
Mean of three studies	31±3	6.1	150	20
Butter beans,	30±2	5.9	150	20
Chickpeas, dried	31	9.2	150	30
Chickpeas	33	.8	150	30
Mean of four studies	28±6	8.3	150	30
Chickpeas, canned	42	9.4	150	22
Chickpeas, curry	41	6.7	150	16
Haricot/Navy beans	39	11.6	150	30
Navy beans second highest GL				
Mean of five studies	38±6	11.8	150	31
Kidney/white bean,	13	3.2	150	25
Kidney beans	23	5.7	150	25
Kidney beans red	25	6.2	150	25
Kidney beans, dried	42	10.3	150	25
Mean of eight studies	28±4	6.9	150	25
Kidney beans, canned	52	9.0	150	17
Black bean	0	4.9	150	25
Mean of two studies	29±1	5.2	150	18
Lentils, green,	52	9.0	150	17
Lentils, red,	18	3.3	150	18
Lentils, red,	32	5.9	150	18
Mean of four studies	26±4	4.8	150	18
Lima beans, baby	32	9.6	150	30

Food:	GI	GL	Serving gm	Carbs gm
Pigeon Pea	22	4.4	150	20
Pinto beans, dried,	39	10.0	150	26
Pinto beans,	45	9.8	150	22
Romano beans	46	8.4	150	18
Soya beans, dried	15±5	0.9	150	6
Soya beans, dried	20±3	1.2	150	6
Mean of two studies	18±3	1.1	150	6
Soya beans, canned	14±2	0.8	150	6
Split peas, yellow	32	6.1	150	19
Cashew nuts, salted	22±5	2.8	50	13
Peanuts (Canada)6	13±6	0.9	50	7
Mean of three studies	14±8	0.8	50	6
Popcorn, microwave	55±7	5.9	20	11
Popcorn, microwave	89	9.6	20	11
Popcorn without butter				
Pea, frozen, boiled	51±6	3.6	80	7
Pea, green	54±14	3.8	80	7
Mean of three studies	48±5	3.4	80	7
Pumpkin	75±9	3.3	80	4
Sweet corn on cob,	48	7.6	80	16
Sweet corn,	60	10.7	80	18
Mean of six studies	54±4	9.3	80	17
Beetroot	64±16	4.6	80	7
Carrots, raw	16	1.2	80	8
Carrots, boiled	49±2	2.2	80	5
Mean of four studies	47±16	2.7	80	6
Cassava, boiled	46	12.0	100	27
Parsnips	97±19	12.1	80	12
Potato ALL POTATOES		>10		
Sweet potato/yam		>13		
Avoid potatoes				
Swede (rutabaga)	72±8	7.5	150	10
Tapioca boiled	81	14.2	250	18
Tapioca, steamed	70±10	12.3	250	18

Tables are available at http://www.glycemicindex.com

Energy density: Foods, which have a low glycemic load, have low energy per unit mass. One way to express this is energy density (ED). Look at calories per gram and calculate the energy density from the known calorie tables or food labels. At the top of the food label ED= calories per serving divided by grams per serving. This can be helpful if you do not have the glycemic index available to calculate a glycemic load. Moreover, ED can be calculated for fats, proteins, as well as complex foods. Just take the calories and divide by the grams from the food label. The table below shows an example of energy density for different foods.

Energy Density = calories/ grams.

	GI	GL	Grams	Carb	CAL/g	ED
Cornflakes:	92	23.9	30g	26	100/28g	3.57
Wheat bread:	73	10.1	30g	14	69/28.3	2.44
Bacon:			100g		500/100	5.0
Chicken:			100g		200/100	2.0

A slice of whole wheat bread and chicken would be a better choice

Studies by B. Rolls at the Pennsylvania State University showed that when the portion size or energy density was reduced it resulted in a reduction in energy intake. A decrease in 25% portion size led to a 10% decrease in energy intake and a decrease in 25% energy density led to a 24% decrease in energy intake. This was measured as 231 calories plus 575 calories respectively. That is in excess of a pound a week of loss on ED reduction alone! In both lean and obese women, changing the energy density resulted in lower energy intake than lowering the fat content.

Since GL and ED are underpinnings of the Food Wheel, following the wheel results in low glycemic load and low energy density consumption.

Satiety: Hunger is one of the strongest and most beneficial stimuli. It helps insure that enough energy for your need is consumed. However, it also works against you when you are trying to lose weight. You could easily lose weight just by eating less. However, the less you eat or the longer you postpone eating, the hungrier you become and the longer it takes your hunger to subside. The hungrier you are, the more you will eat, and your weight loss reverses. Eating provides satiety, a pleasant feeling of fullness, and a corresponding reduction of hunger.

Foods that contain large amounts of fat, sugar, and/or starch have low satiety and are much easier to overeat. Foods that contain large amounts of water, dietary fiber, and/or protein such as fruits have the highest satiety. High satiety includes most vegetables, fruits, and lean meats.

Satiety Index of Some Common Foods

Banana	2.5	**Bean sprouts**	4.6
Macaroni and cheese	2.5	**Watermelon**	4.5
Spaghetti	2.2	**Grapefruit**	4.0
White rice	2.1	**Carrots**	3.8
Pizza	2.1	**Oranges**	3.5
Peanuts	2.0	**Fish, broiled**	3.4
Ice cream	1.8	**Chicken**	3.3
White bread	1.8	**Apples**	3.3
Raisins	1.6	**Sirloin steak**	3.2
Snickers Bar	1.5	**Oatmeal**	3.0
Honey	1.4	**Popcorn**	2.9
Sugar (sucrose)	1.3	Baked potato	2.5

The food Wheel encourages foods with a high satiation index greater than 2.5, low energy density less than 2, and low glycemic load less than 10.

A NEW PARADIGM: THE FOOD WHEEL

A number of problems with the USDA Food Pyramids have been pointed out in the literature:

1. The USDA triangle erroneously promotes the idea that all fats are bad and all carbohydrates are good.
2. By grouping all fats and oils together with sweets, the difference between good fats (unsaturated) and bad fats (saturated and Trans unsaturated fatty acids) are not distinguished.
3. Proteins like meat, poultry, fish, beans, eggs, and nuts are lumped together without noting their many differences.
4. Potatoes/yams, a high glycemic load starch, are not differentiated from other vegetables.
5. There is no differentiation between low-fat and high-fat dairy products.
6. Bread, cereal, rice, and pasta are grouped together without noting differences in GI and GL.
7. The USDA Food Pyramid reflects intensive food industry lobbying not good nutrition science.
8. It is difficult to portray the difference between the qualities/quantities of foods in each food group in a triangular presentation.
9. Placement of foods at the base or apex is meant to imply eat more at the base and less at the apex, which may not be appropriate for all foods because there are some in each group that need emphasis.
10. Something pragmatic is needed that can provide a daily reference for food choices.

Evidence now indicates that not all fats are bad, energy dense carbohydrates (high glycemic load) promote poor glycemic control, and resting energy expenditure increases less with the low glycemic load diet. The National Heart, Lung, and Blood Institute conducted two key studies: Dietary Approaches to Stop Hypertension (DASH) and DASH-Sodium studies. These studies used an eating plan that is low in saturated fat, cholesterol, dairy fat, salt, red meats, and sweets. The plan retains the idea of servings of each food group. The DASH Diet emphasized consumption of low energy-dense fruits and vegetables as its foundation. There is a lack of differentiation or definition of sweets, oils, and grains. A potato produces glucose +glucose and sugar produces glucose + fructose. Therefore, a potato is sweeter than sugar and should be at the apex. Oils are grouped together and are positioned as less preferable than red meat. DASH also recommends 7-8 servings of grains per day. The glycemic load of grains is generally greater than 10.

Patients on the DASH diet showed lowered blood pressure and LDL cholesterol and homocysteine. The USDA 2006 recommendations have included the DASH diet. The new USDA Mypyramid still emphasizes that all carbohydrates are good and all fats are bad but allows DASH food choices.

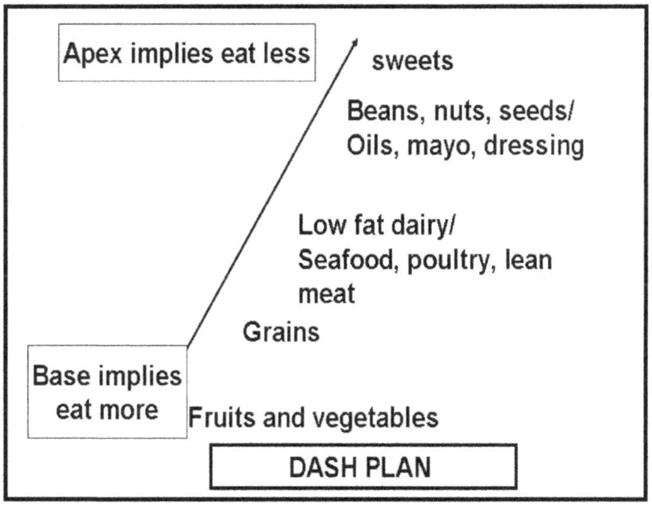

Actual DASH Pyramid available at http://www.nhlbi.nih.gov/health/public/heart/hbp/dash/

The American Heart Association has had a great impact on the American diet by influencing the medical community and by influencing the nutrition standards promoted by the USDA. Remember the "Heart Healthy" food labels. The AHA is promoting low fat consumption. Their guidelines are not easily used by the average citizen. Limiting your trans fat to less than 10 percent of your total calories may not be practical advice unless you are tracking everything eat.

AHA Recommendations

Eat at least five daily servings of fruit and vegetables.

Eat at least six daily servings of grain & whole grains.

Eat at least two servings of oily fish per week.

Eat 25-30 grams of fiber per day.

Limit cholesterol to less than 300 mg a day and less than 200 mg a day for those with heart disease risk factors.

Limit saturated fat and trans fat to less than 10 percent of total calories. Select fats and oils with two grams or less saturated fat per tablespoon.

Limit salt intake to less than six grams (2,300 mg sodium).

If you drink, limit alcohol consumption to no more than one drink per day for women and two drinks per day for men.

Balance the number of calories you eat with the number you use each day.

Several efforts have been made to produce a revised food pyramid. Donald Hensrud, MD from the Mayo Clinic proposed a new healthy eating pyramid to encourage weight loss. The Mayo Clinic pyramid focuses on consumption of unlimited amount of vegetables and fruits in order to decrease energy dense foods, certain carbohydrates, and take the emphasis off counting calories. Mayo Clinic pyramid places fruits and vegetables at its base and encourages consumption of heart-healthy monounsaturated fats. Physical activity is central to the plan. Oils, sweets, and carbohydrates are not differentiated.

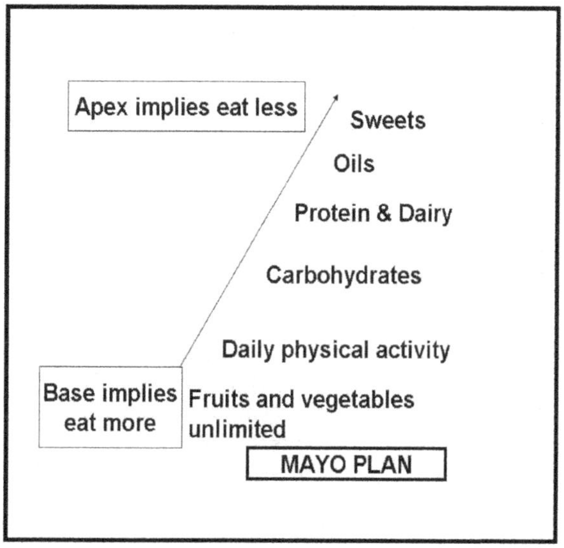

Actual Mayo pyramid can be viewed at http://www.mayoclinic.org/news2000-rst/772.html

Demographic studies of diets indigenous to different societies were done by Oldways Preservation Trust (a Boston based educational organization) indicated as it did for Ansel Keys that certain countries had a high correlation of coronary artery disease (CAD) and fat consumption. However, when the kinds of fats were factored in, different results were appreciated. The fat consumption of Mediterranean countries was just as high as or greater than other countries. However, the fats were predominately vegetables oils. The incidence of heart disease in Mediterranean countries was significantly less because the high consumption of omega 3 and omega 6 oils.

In January 1993, the Harvard University School of Public Health and Oldways Preservation & Exchange held a conference on the Mediterranean diet and its impact on public health. They reviewed data from a variety of epidemiological studies that described the dietary traditions of the people from the Mediterranean area (Crete, Greece, Southern Italy, and Northern Africa) which may be responsible for the low rates of chronic disease. This distinction has resulted in the Mediterranean diet.

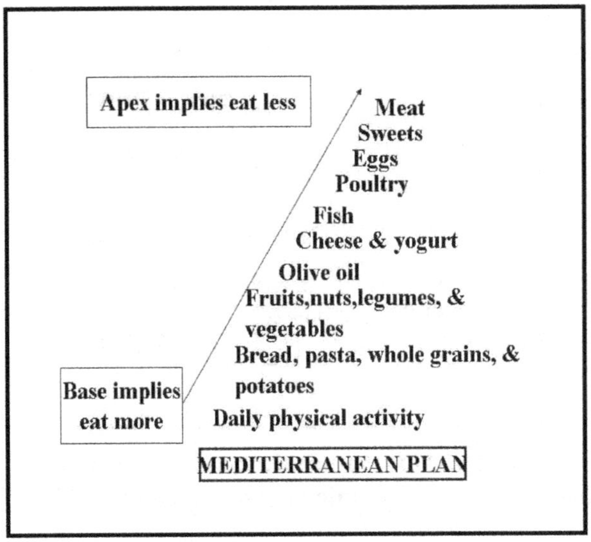

The Mediterranean Pyramid can be viewed at http://www.oldwayspt.org/

The Mediterranean plan emphasizes foods eaten in Mediterranean countries:

1. Abundance of food from plant sources.
2. Emphasis on fresh unprocessed foods.
3. Use olive oil to replace fats.
4. Consumption of low to moderate amount of low fat dairy.
5. Weekly consumption of fish and poultry.
6. Eggs 0-4/week.

7. Fresh fruit as daily dessert snack.
8. Lean red meats (12-16 oz) few times per month.
9. Regular physical activity.
10. Moderate consumption of red wine.

High glycemic load whole grains and potatoes remain a recommended daily consumption.

More importantly is the concept of glycemic index and glycemic load. GI/GL is positively associated with the risk of obesity, insulin resistance, and Diabetes. Dr David Ludwig from Children's Hospital in Boston, an extensive researcher on glycemic index, has characterized a food pyramid based on the glycemic index. We can see here that the grains, potatoes, sweets, and grains are discouraged and fruits and vegetables are encouraged with proteins in moderation.

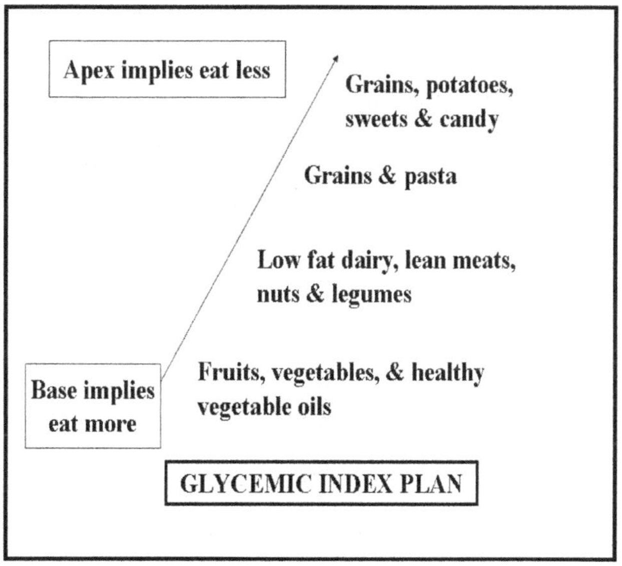

The GI Pyramid can be reviewed at http://www.childrenshospital.org/dream/DreamWin04/how.html

The Researchers at Harvard School of Public Health have developed an alternative to the USDA Food Pyramid, which emphasizes food with low glycemic load and heart healthy fats. More than 50,000 men and 90,000 women were followed 10 to 15 years in the Health Professionals Follow-up Study and the Nurses' Health Study. Researchers found that men who followed the Harvard Healthy Eating Pyramid lowered overall risk of major chronic disease by 20%, and women lowered their overall risk by 11% as compared to the USDA pyramid. The Harvard plan is the more complex in that it tries to differentiate between and within food groups.

We see that vegetable oils have become desirable. Red met and carbohydrates have become undesirable. Carbohydrates are split between whole grains and white carbohydrates. Nuts and legumes are part of the proteins with fish, eggs, and lean meats. Physical activity is a basic element.

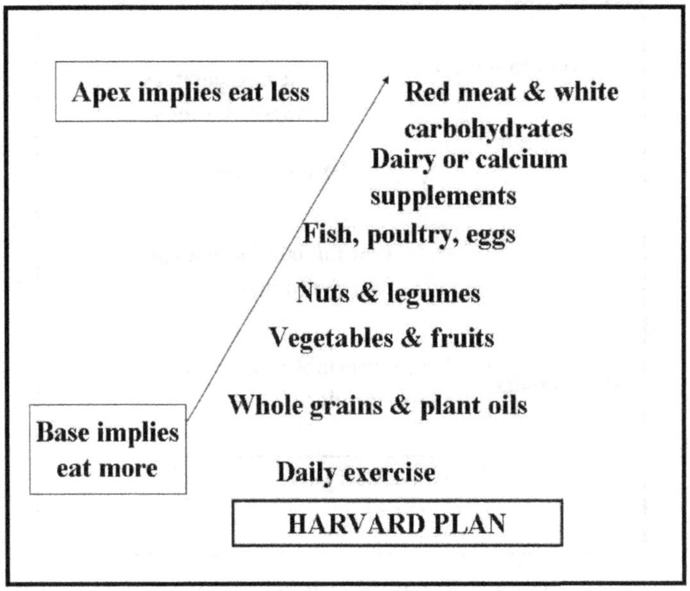

Harvard Pyramid can be viewed at http://www.hsph.harvard.edu/nutritionsource/pyramids.html

It becomes apparent that the choice of a healthy eating plan must incorporate proper nutrition for heart healthy omega fats, low animal cholesterol, low glycemic load carbohydrates, low energy density, and high satiety foods.

A new paradigm is needed to delineate food groups, recommend level of consumption, point out foods to avoid, and provide a pragmatic pictorial. That new paradigm is The Food Wheel.

HEALTHY EATING FOOD WHEEL

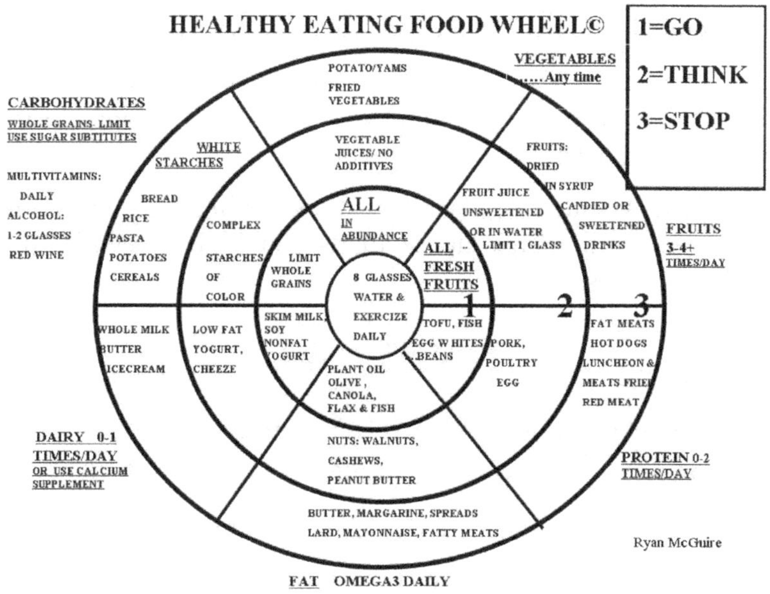

Cumulatively, the data represents a significant paradigm shift away from the USDA Food Pyramid model. Not all fats are bad and not all carbohydrates are good. A new wheel presentation incorporates the concept of low GL, low energy density, high satiety, and the ideas of the DASH, Harvard, Mediterranean, and Mayo Clinic pyramids. The Food Wheel provides a quick flexible reference to determine preferable foods, foods that should be eaten in moderation, and foods that should be avoided within each group and can be tailored to individual energy needs.

EXPLORING THE FOOD WHEEL

Starting from the center, we will explore each section of the food wheel. The top half of the circle refers to your blood sugar, the bottom half refers to your fats and proteins. Together, they are the total **ENERGY YOU CONSUME**.

1= GREEN: You can eat these all the time because the glycemic load is low and energy density is low.

2= YELLOW: Be cautious, eat sometimes. Remember you are trying to lower your total energy as well. Return to the green for snacks.

3=RED: Avoid or eat sparingly, they are high in undesirable fats, salt, and energy dense foods and high glycemic load carbohydrates.

Food Wheel Rules

- Drink eight glasses of water every day.
- Daily, exercise to your capacity.
- For weight maintenance calories = weight x 12.
- Reduce daily intake by 500 calories if BMI >25.
- Eat fresh fruits and vegetables any time.
- Limit sodium to 2000 mg a day.
- Limit sweet drinks, juice, and high fructose corn syrup.
- Avoid white carbohydrates, GL >10.
- Avoid solid fats. Use Canola or fish oil high in omega 3.
- Foods in a bag, box, or can have extra salt, sugar, or fat.
- Eat vegetables raw anytime. Not potatoes or yams.

- Choose only one dairy/hormone/lactase product a day.
- May consume one or two glasses of red wine daily.
- Multivitamins with minerals for most over 50 years old.
- Choose lean meats such as poultry and fish.
- Choose foods with energy density (ED) of 2 or less.
- Advertised high fiber foods contain considerable carbohydrates, salt, and fat.
- Use the Food wheel to guide food purchase.
- Read the USDA food labels; the rest is advertisement, not health information.
- Every thing you buy you will eventually eat.
- Extra energy consumed is extra energy conserved.

Water: Water, at the center of the Food Wheel, is crucial to your health. It makes up, on average, 60 percent of your body weight. Every system in your body depends on water. Lack of water can lead to dehydration. Even mild dehydration of one percent to two percent loss of your body weight can sap your energy and make you tired. Dehydration poses a particular health risk for the very young and the very old. Every day you lose water through sweating (noticeable and unnoticeable) exhaling, urinating, and bowel movements. For your body to function properly, you need to replace this water by consuming beverages and foods that contain water. So how much water, or more precisely fluid, do you need? A healthy adult's daily fluid intake can vary widely. Most people drink fluid to quench thirst to supply perceived water needs.

At least three approaches estimate total fluid (water) needs for healthy, sedentary adults living in a temperate climate.

The replacement approach is based on fluids you loose. The average urine output for adults is 1.5 liters a day. You lose close to an additional liter of water a day through breathing, sweating, and bowel movements. Food usually accounts for 20 percent of your fluid intake. If you consume

2 liters of liquid a day (about 8 cups), along with your normal diet, you will replace the lost fluids.

Another approach to water intake is the 8 x 8 rule. Drink eight 8-ounce glasses of water/fluid a day (about 1.9 liters). Though this approach is not supported by scientific evidence, many people use this basic rule as a guideline for how much fluid to drink.

The Institute of Medicine recommends that men consume 3 liters (about 13 cups) of total beverages a day and women consume 2.2 liters (about 9 cups) of total beverages a day. These guidelines are based on national food surveys that assessed people's average fluid intakes.

You can choose any of these fluid intake approaches to gauge your fluid needs. However, your current total fluid intake is probably sufficient if you drink enough water to quench your thirst and produce a colorless or slightly yellow normal amount of urine. You may need to increase total fluid intake from these recommended amounts depending on several factors, including how active you are, the climate, your health status, age greater than 70, and if you're pregnant or breast-feeding. If you exercise or engage in any activity that makes you sweat, you will need to drink extra water to compensate for that fluid loss. Your diet can provide a large portion of what you need. In an average adult food provides about 20 percent of total water intake.

Beware of liquid candy. According to the National Soft Drink Association (NSDA), the consumption of soft drinks is now over 600 12-ounce servings (12 oz.) per person per year. Since 1978, soda consumption in the US has tripled for boys and doubled for girls. Young males age 12-29 are the biggest consumers at over 160 gallons per year-that is almost 2 quarts per day. At these levels, the calories from soft drinks can contribute as much as 10 percent of the total daily caloric intake. High Fructose Corn Syrup (HFCS), now used in preference to sugar, is associated with poor development of collagen in growing animals, especially in the context of copper deficiency. The liver must metabolize fructose. Therefore, high fructose consumption promotes liver changes similar to those of alcoholics. Aspartame, used in diet sodas, is a potent neurotoxin and endocrine disrupter. Caffeine stimulates the adrenal gland without providing nourishment. In large amounts, caffeine can lead to adrenal exhaustion in children. Phosphoric acid is associated with calcium loss. Citric acid and artificial flavors often contains traces of MSG, a neurotoxin.

Make a conscious effort to keep yourself hydrated by choosing water as your beverage of choice. This is central to the Food Wheel.

Exercise: Exercise is central to health and is at the center of the Food Wheel. Walking is a natural motion that requires little skill or athletic ability and is therefore the ideal exercised for many people. Daily walking or regular aquatic exercises can strengthen the heart, help in weight control, build endurance, and reduce mental stress. Both place little physical stress on the joints and making injury less likely than with other activities. Walking, in addition, does not require a partner or special facility. Research has shown that the greatest health benefits of exercise occur when sedentary people become moderately active.

Always start slowly. Many people make the mistake of trying to do too much too soon. It is very important to start slowly in order to avoid injury and prevent burnout. The speed and duration of your walking session should depend on your initial degree of fitness. Start low, go slow, and keep a record of your progress.

Always warm up. A warm-up should include a 5-minute slow walk to increase blood flow to exercising muscles. After this low intensity walk, stretch all the major muscle groups of the body paying special attention to the muscles of the legs and hips to prevent stiffness and therefore prevent injuries. As a rule of thumb, if you cannot carry on a conversation while you are walking you may be going too fast.

Always cool down. A proper cool down includes a slow walk and stretching. The slow walk prevents blood from pooling in the legs. Stretching after exercise helps maintain flexibility and prevents cramping. Accumulating thirty minutes of walking five days of the week is enough activity to elicit many health benefits.

Initiating strenuous exercise when you have existing risks such as high blood pressure, diabetes, heart problems, or breathing problems should require a medical clearance and possibly an exercise stress test.

Carbohydrates: The top half of the food wheel contains macronutrients that are composed predominantly of carbohydrates. The pie section label for carbohydrates is red, which cautions us to stop! Starch and cellulose are two common carbohydrates. Both are macromolecules with molecular weights in the hundreds of thousands. Cellulose is fiber and cannot be digested by the human body. The links that compose both starch and cellulose are units of sugar.

Monosaccharides are three common single sugars that share the same molecular formula $C_6H_{12}O_{6:}$ Glucose is the human body's source of energy transported by blood. Galactose is a sugar in milk products. Fructose is a sugar found in honey and fruit. Two monosaccharides can be linked together to form a double sugar or disaccharide. Three common disaccharides are Sucrose (common table sugar = glucose + fructose), lactose (major sugar in milk = glucose + galactose), maltose (product of starch digestion = glucose + glucose. Note that potato maltose starch is sweeter than sugar.

All sugars are very soluble in water. Sugars are the most important source of energy. Carbohydrates provide the bulk of the calories (4 kcal/gram) in most diets, and starches provide the bulk of the carbohydrates. Starches are polysaccharides built from repeating units of glucose much as a chain built from its links. Two types are amylose consisting of linear unbranched chains of several hundred glucose units and amylopectin consisting of several thousand highly branched chains.

Starches are insoluble in water and can serve as storage depots of glucose. Plants convert excess glucose into starch for storage. Rice, wheat, and potatoes are major sources of starch in the human diet. Before starches can enter or leave cells, they must be broken down with water (hydrolysis). This converts it into glucose. Animals store excess glucose by polymerizing it to form glycogen. The structure of glycogen is similar to that of a starch, although the branches in glycogen tend to be shorter and more frequent. Glycogen is broken back down into glucose when energy is needed (a process called glycogenolysis). Major depots of glycogen stores are the liver (20%) and skeletal muscles (80%). Excess energy is converted to fat.

Here are some cautions when choosing carbohydrates:

- Choose foods that use the word "whole" first on the label's ingredient list. Eat in moderation because whole grain products can have a significant glycemic load.
- Foods labeled with the words "multi-grain," "stone-ground," "100% wheat," "cracked wheat," "seven-grain," or "bran" are usually not whole-grain products.
- Color is not an indication of a whole grain.
- Use the Nutrition Facts label and choose products with a higher percentage Daily Value (%DV) for fiber.
- Read the food label's ingredient list. Look for terms that indicate added sugars (sucrose, high-fructose corn syrup, honey, and molasses) and oils (partially hydrogenated vegetable oils) that add extra calories.

All wheat-products like bread, pasta, pizza, cookies, cake, and pastries contain opioid peptides. One wheat-gluten protein-molecule contains a number of extremely powerful opioid peptides. Some of these molecules are even 100 times more powerful than a morphine molecule. Examples are Glycine-Tyrosine-Tyrosine-Proline, Tyrosine-Glycine-Glycine-Tryptophane, Tyrosine-Proline-Isoleucine-Serine-Leucine, Tyrosine-Glycine-Glycine-

Tryptophane-Leucine, and Tyrosine-Glycine-Glycine (endorphin related). To compensate the analgesic effect wheat products often contain rosemarin extract.

The Roman rulers already new the people would not rise against them as long as they were entertained and fed bread.

The Food Wheel cautions us to avoid white refined energy dense carbohydrates and eat whole grain foods in moderation only. If it is in a bag, box, or can it probably will contain something you should not consume.

Fruits and Vegetables: The other two pie sections of the top half of the Food Wheel are fruits and vegetables. Vegetables are nature's natural carbohydrates, which contain vitamins, minerals, and have a low Glycemic Load. Potatoes and yams are the exception. Snacking on low-calorie, fiber-rich fruits and vegetables help keep both calories and hunger in check. Vitamins, minerals, fiber, and protective substances called phytochemicals found in fruits and vegetables, help prevent cancer by neutralizing harmful by-products of metabolism inside cells. Other phytochemicals appear to help detoxify carcinogens and block cancer growth. Fruits and vegetables are naturally low in sodium, rich in potassium, and virtually fat free. Many also provide a healthy dose of foliate and carotenoids. According to a report by the American Institute for Cancer Research, if everyone consumed a diet rich in fruits and vegetables, 20 percent or more of all cases of cancers could be prevented. A diet rich in fruits and vegetables is associated with a lower risk of stroke, cataracts, diverticulosis, improved blood lipid levels, and a longer life.

Care needs to be taken when consuming fruit and vegetable juices. Many contain considerable additives in addition to sugars, fructose, and salt. Juices should be limited to a glass a day. Read the food label carefully.

The top portion of the Food Wheel tells us to avoid excessive carbohydrates from processed foods and white starches. Eat whole grains in moderation. Nature's

natural carbohydrates are fruits and vegetables. Return to them for snacks. Limit juices to one glass a day. Processed foods are a recent addition to the human diet. Our Paleolithic ancestors show us that we are not compatible with processed foods.

Lipids: Fat has a bad reputation. Thanks to Ansel Keys and the American Heart Association, it is a word associated with obesity, heart disease, and many other disease states. However, not all fats are bad fats. The different types of dietary fat fall into three main groups: saturated, mono-unsaturated, and polyunsaturated fat. Saturated fats are the animal-derived 'hard' fats such as butter, lard, fat in meat, and those used in processed foods. Saturated fats are a chain of carbon atoms jointed by single links, which means that the maximum amount of hydrogen is present. These are the kind of fats you need to avoid in your eating plan. Of the unsaturated fats, monounsaturated fatty acids (MUFA) are made up of a chain of carbon atoms containing one double bond. They characteristically have a lower melting point than saturated fats and so are generally liquids (oils) rather than solids (fats). Olive oil is the best-known example of oil, which contains predominantly monounsaturated fatty acids. A polyunsaturated fatty acid (PUFA) has more than one double bond in the chain. Vegetable oils such as canola oil and the oils from fish contain high levels of polyunsaturates. Polyunsaturated fatty acids are further divided into two sub-groups called omega-6 and omega-3. Both the omega-6 and omega-3 fatty acids belong to a group of polyunsaturated fats called 'essential' because they are necessary to life and to health and they must be obtained from diet. The omega-3s have anti-inflammatory benefits and help prevent heart disease, whereas omega-6s lower blood cholesterol and support the skin. Both of these groups are essential for good health and normal growth.

For most of the time humans have been on earth, we have eaten foods containing omega-6s and omega-3s in a ratio of about 2:1. The human diet today is vastly different from that of our ancestors even a few hundred years ago. In fact, the greatest diet changes have occurred in the past 50 years. Our increasing reliance on cereals, processed foods, vegetable oils, and spreads, has resulted in a ratio of omega-6/omega-3 in the USA is around 12:1 Modern Western diets are deficient in omega-3 fatty acids. With simple measures, you can make a big difference. Cut down on fried foods and use canola for cooking and in salad dressings. Avoid soft margarines (made from sunflower, safflower, or Soya). Reduce consumption of processed foods, as these are normally high in saturated or omega-6 fats. Increase consumption of fish or fish oil supplement. Aim for a regime that supplies a minimum 1000mg omega-3 a day. You can obtain omega-3 from sources such as flaxseed (linseed) oil, walnuts and walnut oil, rapeseed (canola) oil, chia seeds, and dark green leafy vegetables. Fish supplies the preferred omega-3 already converted as eicosapentaenoic acid and docosahexaenoic acid (EPA and DHA) that the body can use most readily. Because the omega-3 and omega-6 compete on the same metabolic pathway, excessive omega-6 may block conversion of omega-3 ALA to the more useful omega-3 EPA and DHA. Nonfish eaters must be extra vigilant in cutting down on excess omega-6 intake. The following levels represent typical values of the most commonly consumed oil-rich fish.

<u>Grams of Omega-3 per 100g of Fish</u>

Sprat	2. 4	Tuna (fresh or frozen)	1. 6
Salmon	2. 3	Anchovy	1. 4
Sardine/pilchard	2. 2	Crab	1. 2
Mackerel	2. 0	Rainbow trout	1. 2
Herring	1. 6	Shrimp (boiled)	0. 8

The three predominant meats in the west are beef, chicken, and pork. The following table shows that the inherent inclusion of fat in the beef muscle bundles causes beef to be fatter per gram than any other meat.

Comparison of fats in Beef, Chicken, and Pork

Per 100g raw weight	**Lean Pork**	**Skinless chicken breast**	**Lean beef**
Energy (kJ)	440	440	610
Protein (g)	22.2	22.3	22.5
Total fats (g)	1.2	1.6	6.0

Your doctor may order a lipid panel, also called a lipid profile, which usually includes four measurements of the types of fats (lipids) in your blood:

Low-density lipoprotein (LDL) cholesterol is sometimes called the bad cholesterol because too much of it in your blood causes the accumulation of fatty deposits (plaques) in your arteries (atherosclerosis), reducing blood flow and leading to heart disease. In addition, in people with diabetes, LDL cholesterol molecules tend to be smaller and denser than in people without diabetes, causing further damage to blood vessels. A 10 percent reduction in LDL level would drop the rate of heart disease by 30 percent.

High-density lipoprotein (HDL) cholesterol is sometimes called the "good" cholesterol because it helps carry LDL cholesterol back to your liver and keep arteries open. Triglycerides help your body store fat. Total cholesterol is a sum of your cholesterol content.

Although these lipids are necessary for your body to function normally, the kind and amount present in your blood might indicate if you are at increased risk of heart disease. Together, the four numbers can provide clues about your risk of having a heart attack, stroke, or other blood vessel damage (vascular disease). All adults should have a fasting lipoprotein profile done every 5 years.

How dietary fats effect your blood cholesterol			
Type of Fat	Main Source	State at Room Temp	Effect on Levels: LDL=BAD HDL= GOOD
Monounsaturated Canola, flaxseed oil Highest in omega 3	Olives; olive oil, canola oil, peanut oil; cashews, almonds, peanuts, and most other nuts; avocados	Liquid	Lowers LDL; raises HDL
Polyunsaturated Fish high in omega 3	Corn, soybean, safflower, and cottonseed oils; fish	Liquid	Lowers LDL; raises HDL
Saturated	Whole milk, butter, cheese, and ice cream; red meat; chocolate; coconuts, and coconut oil	Solid	Raises LDL and HDL
Trans	margarines; vegetable shortening; partially hydrogenated vegetable oil; deep-fried chips; baked goods	Solid or semi-solid	Raises LDL

Nuts contain heart healthy omega 3 oils. The Nurse's Health Study, including 86,016 women followed for 14 years, showed women who ate five or more ounces of nuts a week reduced their risk of death from heart attacks by 35 percent. This reduction continued even after adjusting for obesity, blood pressure, exercise, smoking, alcohol, vitamin E, dietary fats, dietary fiber, red meat, fruit, and vegetable intake. In non-smokers and nondrinkers, the frequent nut users reduced their risk by 52 percent. In the Iowa Women's Health Study, women who ate nuts frequently, compared to those who seldom ate nuts, reduced their risk of fatal heart disease by 57 percent. Here are a few of the reasons researchers believe nuts are good for your health:

1. Although nuts are high in fat, the fat is mostly unsaturated fat, which has a beneficial effect on health.
2. Almonds and walnuts have both shown a beneficial effect on blood cholesterol levels.
3. The protein in nuts is high in arginine, a precursor to nitric oxide, which is important to help keep blood vessels relaxed and open and helps prevent clotting.
4. Walnuts in particular, are high in alpha-linolenic acid, an essential (n-3 or omega) fatty acid that is protective to the heart and circulation. This fat has been shown to reduce the risk of heart disease and fatal arrhythmias in various studies.
5. Nuts are also good sources of dietary fiber, magnesium, copper, folic acid, vegetable protein, potassium, and vitamin E, all of which have been shown to be important for heart health.

Plant sterols/stanols are similar in chemical structure to cholesterol. They are found naturally in a range of plant sources such as vegetable oils, nuts, grains, seeds, wood pulp, and leaves. Foods supplemented with plant sterols/stanols may reduce cholesterol and are a promising addition to interventions aimed at lowering heart disease risk. Plant sterols are thought to decrease the absorption of dietary and derived cholesterol in the gut. The FDA has approved the following health claim for plant stanol/sterol esters and reduced risk of heart disease: Diets low in saturated fat and cholesterol that include at least 1.3 grams of plant sterol esters or 3.4 grams of plant stanol esters, consumed in two meals with other foods, may reduce the risk of heart disease. Available spreads are Benecol, Pro Active, and Take Control. Most trials of the plant sterol enriched foods which show that they do have an effect on blood cholesterol do not directly compare eating these products with eating a healthy diet rich in fruit and vegetables, although the companies state that the benefits of the products are found when eaten as part of a healthy diet and lifestyle.

There is a counter position to the lipid hypothesis. In the early 1900, Russian researchers noted that feeding rabbits, cholesterol (animal fat) caused a build-up of fatty deposits in their arteries. Rabbits are not metabolically equipped to eat animal products. Scientists began examining possible links between fat, cholesterol, and coronary heart disease in humans. Ancel Keys plotted the coronary heart disease (CHD) death rates from seven (selected) country studies of diet and heart disease and showed a correlation between fat consumption and CHD. However, mortality data available for all the 22 countries did not support his hypothesis. The American Heart Association noted that the American daily consumption of energy was 40% fat and CHD was dramatically increasing. Lipid theories were officially incorporated into AHA dietary guideline. The lipid hypothesis evolved into a central fixture of mainstream health policy where it was incorporated into the USDA food pyramid in 1962. Here are the cholesterol ideas that have been propagated:

1. Cholesterol is a deadly poison. Actually, it is a vital substance necessary for cells of all animals.

2. High blood cholesterol causes atherosclerosis and coronary disease. Many studies have shown that people with low lipids have atherosclerosis. There has not been a single controlled clinical trial that has shown any reduction in coronary heart disease (CHD) mortality attributed to lowering of cholesterol.
3. Diet can lower cholesterol. Our bodies produce three to four times more cholesterol than we eat. The production changes inversely to the amount we eat. Therefore, diet can change only a few percent.
4. Heart mortality and total mortality has been improved with cholesterol drugs. The only effective way to lower cholesterol is with drugs but mortality has not been shown to improve.
5. The new statin drugs improve cardiovascular disease by lowering cholesterol. Actually, they act as antioxidants. This has been in evidence concerning homocystine-promoting oxidation of LDL cholesterol.
6. Drug companies selling lipid lowering statin drugs have funded the majority of money spent on lipid research.
7. If new recommendations were implemented, about 4,000,000 persons would be added to those already taking statin drugs. (What a bonanza for drug company profits). Six out of the nine members of the National Cholesterol Education Program (NCEP) making these new recommendations are affiliated with the drug companies that manufacture statin drugs.
8. Dr. Kilmer McCulley gets credit for discovering the critical role of homocysteine. Homocysteine stops the production of the valuable vasodilating nitric acid, causes blood to thicken, and facilitates the oxidation of LDL cholesterol, thus setting the stage for atherosclerotic plaque and blood clots to form. High homocysteine levels cause cholesterol to change to

oxidized low-density lipoprotein, which damages the arteries. Most people do not get enough folic acid, vitamin B_6, or vitamin B_{12} in their diet. Recent studies indicate that homocysteine may just be a marker not a cause.

The Food Wheel tells us that consumption of lean meats, nuts, canola and flaxseed oils, fish, fish oil, B6, B12, and folic acid promotes cardio health.

Dairy: Goats were domesticated around 7000 B.C. and cattle around 6000 B.C. One of the earliest milking scenes shows a goat being milked on an Elamite seal from 2500 B.C. European dairy cows arrived in America in 1611. Originally, cattle served a triple-purpose: meat, milk, and labor. By the 5th century A.D., cows and sheep were prized for their milk in Europe. By the 14th century, whole herds of sheep were being milked in Europe but cow's milk soon became more popular than sheep's milk. The first ice cream parlor opened in New York City in 1776. The first regular shipment of milk by rail to New York City was in 1841. The first cheese factory in the United States was built in Oneida County, New York in 1851. Pasteurization made it possible to store and distribute milk. Commercial pasteurization machines were first introduced in 1895. High temperature pasteurization was introduced in 1948. In the 20th Century, the dairy industry evolved due to advances in sanitary on-farm milk storage and efficient transportation to processing and packaging facilities. Therefore, humanoids did not start to drink milk from other animals until almost 5,000 years ago. For over 99% of our existence, we did not regard milk as food for human beings. Why do we so now? In fact, every day the average American consumes dairy products equal to the same cholesterol contained in 53 slices of bacon.

The question that is now posed is whether milk is a suitable food for either adults or children in large amounts. Milk protein requires excessive pancreatic enzymes for digestion of cow hormones, which is compounded by lactose intolerance and allergies. When you use 21 pounds of milk to make a pound of butter, or 10 pounds of milk to make a pound of hard cheese, or 8 pounds of milk to make a pound of sherbet, the bovine hormones are concentrate. IGF-1 growth hormone is the one hormone in the animal kingdom that is identical between species, human and cow. IGF-1 is manufactured and supplemented to cows to increase milk production 20-30% and then passed on to us. This insulin growth factor hormone is a key factor in the growth and proliferation of breast cancer, lung cancer, prostate cancer, and other cancers in humans. In a woman's lifetime, she will produce one tablespoon of estrogen. This means that it takes only a billionth of a gram of cow hormones to produce a powerful biological effect like early sexual maturity in young girls. Men with high IGF-1 are more likely to develop prostate cancer.

Milk also contains opioid peptides. Milk-opioid peptides are beta-casomorphins, alpha-casein exorphins, casoxins, beta-casorphins, alpha-lactorphins, beta-lactorphins, and lactaferroxins. These opioid peptides cause physical dependence in the young to increase milk consumption and promote sleep for rapid development. Unfortunately, adult milk consumers also absorb those opioid peptides.

The pasteurization of milk changes the structure of the milk proteins and valuable enzymes are destroyed. This makes digestion problematical. Calves fed pasteurized milk exclusively die before maturity.

When milk is homogenized, small fat globules surround the xanthine oxidase and it is absorbed intact into your blood stream. There is some evidence that this enzyme increases risks of heart disease.

When we look at nations where milk consumption is high, we find that heart disease, osteoporosis, cancer, diabetes, and asthma are common. Nations where cheese consumption has tripled in the last 30 years, like England and France and Canada and the United States, have a tripling of asthma and breast cancers. The highest rates of breast cancer are in Denmark, Norway, Holland, and Sweden with the highest consumption of milk products. The connection between milk and strong bones has been mischaracterized by the dairy industry. Bone density attained by age 18 usually lasts a lifetime, provided a balanced diet is maintained. Calcium intake alone is not related to bone density. High protein consumption uses calcium to neutralize the metabolic acid produced. Eskimos consume 250-400 gm of protein and over 2,000 mg of calcium a day. Eskimos have the highest rate of osteoporosis in the world! African Bantu women consume 50 gm protein and 450 mg calcium daily and have on average 10 children. They have no osteoporosis. Cultures that have highest protein consumed have increased osteoporosis. In America 74.5% of the dietary calcium is obtained from dairy products. Those same dairy products (labeled by some as liquid meat), paradoxically, promote osteoporosis.

Below are some of the vegetables that have an abundance of calcium. Note that at the end of the table are the amounts of calcium for milk and cheese. Adequate amounts of vegetables are a better source of calcium because all vegetables and legumes contain calcium.

Milligrams of Calcium per 100 Calories of Food

Arugula	1300	Green onions	240
Watercress	800	Okra	213
Turnip greens	650	Cabbage	196
Collard greens	548	American cheese	160
Mustard greens	490	Milk 2%	245
Spinach	450	Swiss cheese	250
Broccoli	387		

Milk and milk-based products can be very healthy for you in moderation. It is not healthy to consume more than a serving of bovine/hormones/ lactose by-product a day. Get your calcium from vegetables. Remember Paleolithic man. Excessive dairy products like excessive carbohydrates are not genetically compatible.

Proteins: Amino acids bond together to create long chains called proteins. Over one hundred amino acids have been found in nature. In Australia, 1969, amino acids were found in the Murchison Meteor, which has been dated at five billion years. Proteins make up about 15% of the mass of the average human body. Muscle, cartilage, ligaments, skin, and hair are all mainly protein materials. There are an estimated 100,000 different proteins in the human body alone, and each of them is made up of different combinations of only twenty-two amino acids. Twenty are standard amino acids, which are encoded by standard genetic code by mRNA translation. There are eight essential amino acids, which cannot be synthesized by the body and must be supplied by consuming proteins in food. Two additional amino acids, histidine and arginine, are essential to children and the elderly. Two additional amino acids, selenocystine and pyrrolysine, are coded by a non-standard pathway.

Protein digestibility and utilization determines the availability of amino acids to produce proteins. Like building blocks, any shortage of a particular essential amino acid results in incomplete protein translation. The residual amino acids are then broken down by the body for energy or converted to lipids. About 1/6 of the amino acids are recycled from the normal degradation of tissue. Muscles are the protein reservoir for the body. Inadequate consumption causes muscle wasting. Over consumption causes acidity, which requires calcium to neutralize, and possible kidney damage.

The daily protein requirement is about 0.8-1.4 grams of protein for each kilogram of body weight. The net protein utilization is profoundly affected by the essential amino acid found in the smallest quantity in each particular food item. The limiting amino acids usually include the sulfur-containing ones (methionine and cysteine), tryptophan, and lysine. Measurement of protein value for human nutrition is done by the protein digestibility-corrected amino acid score (PDCAAS).

There has been concern that vegetarians could not obtain adequate quality or quantity of protein. However, a varied diet will compliment any limited amino acid and supply 100% of requirement.

PDCAAS of common protein sources

Protein source	**Score**
Milk , whey	1.0
Egg white, poultry	1.0
Fish	1.0
Beef	0.92
Nuts	0.7
Legumes, dry beans	0.6
Oats	0.57
Wheat and grains	0.42

Proteins serve two broad purposes in the human body. Structural proteins form most of the solid material in the human body. The structural protein keratin and collagen are the main component of your hair, muscles, tendons, and skin. Functional proteins help carry out activities and functions in the human body. Hemoglobin is a functional protein that occurs in the red blood cells and helps to transport oxygen in the body. Myosin is a protein that is responsible for the ability of muscles to contract.

A sub-class of the functional proteins is enzymes. Enzymes help to carry out specific chemical reactions in the body. For example, amylase is an enzyme that helps to break apart the sugar bonds in the carbohydrate starch. Each protein has a different structure and performs a different function in the body.

The food wheel encourages consumption of non-processed protein sources; choose a variety of lean meats, legumes, nuts, mixed vegetables, and fish.

Fiber: Fiber is an indigestible complex carbohydrate found in various plants. Fiber in itself has no calories because the body cannot absorb it. Fiber can be divided into two categories: water insoluble and water-soluble. Insoluble fibers, such as cellulose, hemicellulose, and lingnin, do not dissolve in water. It is the major structural material which plants are made and probably the single most abundant organic molecule. Soluble fibers, such as gum and pectin dissolve in water. Much research suggests that fiber may prevent cancer, diabetes, heart disease, and obesity. Fiber bulks up wastes and moves it through the colon more rapidly, preventing constipation and possibly colon cancer. Gums and pectins may keep cholesterol under control by removing bile acids that digest fat, slows sugar absorption, and reduces the amount of insulin needed. Clinical reports suggest that soluble fiber (such as psyllium, pectin, and guar gum) may enhance the sensation of fullness and reduce hunger cravings. For these reasons, incorporating soluble fiber such as fiber tabs into the diet may aid weight loss. The average American diet consumes 10-15 grams daily, which is half of the daily goal.

One can substitute commercial sources of fiber. Products such as Metamucil, Hydrocil, Konsyl, Fibercon, and methylcellulose are perfectly good substitute sources of fiber. One tablespoon a day provides 15 grams of the recommended 25-30 grams daily. Additional fiber supplements in the absence of adequate water intake can be binding and cause constipation. There is a necessary balance between fiber content of the diet and water intake.

Cereal Products touted as high fiber, such as cold cereals in the following table, cause rapid rate of increase in blood glucose (GI) and a large quantity of blood glucose (GL). They also can contain significant fat and salt. Do not be fooled by labels such as “heart healthy” and “high fiber”.

Cereal products advertised as high fiber

CEREAL	GI	GL
Bran Flakes	74	13.2
Cheerios™	74	15
Corn Bran™	75	15.2
Corn Chex™	83	20.9
Cornflakes™	92	23.9
Cornflakes, high-fiber	74	16.7
Corn Pops™	80±4	21
Crispix™	87	21.9
Fruit Loops™	69±9	17.9
Frosties™,	55	14.5
Golden Grahams™	71	17.6
Grapenuts™	80	17.4
Life™	66	16
Mini Wheats™,	58±8	12.1
Raisin Bran™	61±5	11.7
Rice Chex™	89	23.3
Rice Krispies™	82	21
Shredded Wheat	75	15
Special K™	69±5	14.3

A prebiotic is defined as a nondigestible food that beneficially affects the host by selectively stimulating the growth and/or activity of one or a limited number of bacteria in the colon. Oligosaccharide refers to a short chain of sugar molecules. Fructo-oligosaccharides (FOS) and inulin consist of short chain fructose molecules and are found in many vegetables. Galacto-oligosaccharides (GOS), which also occurs in mother's milk and initially promotes digestive flora of the new born, consist of short chains of galactose molecules. These compounds can be only partially digested by humans. When oligosaccharides are consumed, the undigested portion serves as food for friendly bacteria in the intestine. The digestive tract is home to more than 400 species of bacteria. Some of these friendly native bugs crowd out invading organisms that cause illness. Inulin, a prebiotic, occurs naturally in large quantities in some of the most famous herbs, such as burdock root, dandelion root, elecampane root, and chicory root. It is soluble only in hot water, and has traditionally been consumed in hot teas. Americans eat less than 3 grams of inulin per day. Sixteenth century Europeans consumed about 35 grams of inulin daily. Europeans of the 19th century consumed up to 100grams daily. This is because of changes in the modern diet, which exclude many natural products in favor of processed foods. The need to include oligosaccharides in our diet is highlighted by scientific studies, which indicate that the human physiological effects of the prebiotic are likely to be:

1. Improved fat metabolism: there is preliminary evidence of a triglyceride-reducing effect of inulin and possible reduction of the risk of colon cancer.
2. Improved bioavailability of minerals such as calcium.
3. Improved bowel functions mainly due to the increase of fecal bulk material.
4. Maintain intestinal flora.
5. Prevent harmful bacteria growth.

A probiotic is defined classically as a viable microbial dietary supplement, such as fermented yogurt containing Bifidobacteria and Lactobacillus species that beneficially affects the host through its effects in the intestinal tract. The bacteria, which are found in probiotic products such as yogurt, kefir, and fermented vegetables usually, are not normally found in the human intestine. In fact, the intestinal environment is often a hostile one for these foreign bacteria. Because of this, bacteria eaten in probiotic products do not colonize the intestine. They are flushed through and eliminated from the body.

The food Wheel makes these points about the consumption of fiber:

1. **The food wheel advises caution when consuming foods advertised as high fiber foods, which can contain significant calories, salt, and fat.**
2. **Increasing the consumption of complex carbohydrates such as fresh fruits and raw or cooked vegetables is the best way to increase fiber intake.**
3. **Substitute legumes for meat. Some, like lentils, are very high in proteins.**
4. **When choosing whole grain foods, the labels must state "whole grain".**
5. **Eat whole fruits instead of drinking fruit juices.**
6. **Read the food label and look for foods with a high percent daily value of fiber (DV%).**
7. **You can choose probiotic fiber tablets before meals with a large glass of water or unsweetened tea to increase satiety, increase fiber intake, and promote healthful intestinal bacteria.**

MICRONUTRIENTS

Vitamins and Minerals: "Vitamine" was the term coined by Casimir Funk (1884-1967) for the unidentified substances present in food, which could prevent the diseases scurvy, beriberi, rickets, and pellagra. Vitamins are essential molecules that act in the regulation of metabolic processes but do not provide energy or serve as building units. The human body needs 13 different vitamins. The U.S. Department of Agriculture studied the diets of a cross section of over 21,000 men and women. They found that not one single person was getting all of the daily requirements of the Recommended Daily Allowance (RDA) from the food they ate. A diet of fruits, vegetables, and meat usually provides all of the vitamins that you need. However, the increased consumption of processed foods results in decreased vitamin intake. Processing tends to destroy vitamins. The RDA is the bare bones minimum amount required to prevent deficiency. The RDA for Vitamin C is only 60 milligrams. Whereas, recent research has set the Optimum Daily Allowance (ODA) for Vitamin C at 500 – 5000 milligrams a day. The ODA protects you from diseases of vitamin deficiency and helps ward off many other diseases. So remember, the ODA is the optimum level of micronutrients necessary to create buoyant, vibrant health. Daily Value (DV) is a government standard that specifies the minimum daily requirements that helps prevent a deficiency disease for healthy people. The DV is based on intake of 2,000 calories per day. If you do intend on having additional supplementation of the antioxidants such as Vitamin C or E it may be advantageous to take these separately. Most of the multi-vitamins do not provide adequate supplemental amounts of these. The chelated (bonding a mineral to an amino acid to make it easier for the body to digest) minerals may be better absorbed because they are protected from substances in foods that can bind with it. For example, the phytic acid in grains or the oxalates in spinach can bind with minerals like calcium, lessening the absorption. Chelated minerals may cost more and claims are not regulated.

In addition, commercial industry uses artificial fertilizers to grow our food. Of the 26 vitamins and minerals essential to human beings, only 17 are necessary for plant growth. Artificial fertilizers, designed to create higher plant yields, overlook the human requirements for these other essential nutrients. This produces nutritionally depleted food. For example, our food has plenty of phosphorus because plants need it. However, plants do not need chromium or selenium to thrive. Therefore, artificial fertilizers may not contain these important minerals. Therefore, our food could be deficient in minerals such as chromium and selenium, which are vitally important to help protect you against cancer, diabetes, and premature aging. Who needs supplements? You may need vitamin or mineral supplementation if you have impaired digestion and absorption of nutrients, eat fewer than 1000 calories per day, limit your diet because of food intolerances, omit all animal products, have poor wound healing, are over 50 years of age, or a high reliance on processed foods.

The Food Wheel recommends a daily multivitamin for those over fifty and to look for the following points:

1. Take 100% of the optimal daily allowances (ODA) for vitamins B1 (thiamin), B2 (riboflavin), niacin (vitamin B6), vitamin B 12, vitamin C, vitamin D, vitamin E, and folic acid.
2. For vitamin A use Beta-carotene which is converted to vitamin A and will not cause vitamin A toxicity.
3. Avoid mega doses of fat-soluble A, D, and E.
4. Do not take the minerals iron, selenium, copper, and zinc long-term unless your medical team recommends it.
5. We get enough phosphorus from our diets, too much can prevent calcium absorption.

6. Iodine, manganese, molybdenum, chloride, and boron are bound to foods and are usually not needed.
7. Look for USP on a label. This specifies that the supplements meet the standards of the U.S. Pharmacopoeia. They have gone through a testing for dissolvability that mimics what happens in your body.
8. Look for the Optimum Daily Allowance range.

Suggested Optimal Daily Nutritional Allowances

Nutrient	**RDA**	**ODA**
Fat-soluble Vitamins		
Vitamin A (I micro gm = 3.33 IU)	800-1,000	2,000
Beta-carotene (mg)	N/A	80-100
Vitamin D (1 microgram = 40 IU)	8- 5	24
Vitamin E (IU) mixed tocopherols	10	800
Vitamin K (mg)	65--80	65--80
Water-soluble Vitamins		
Vitamin C (mg)	60	800--1000
Vitamin B12 (mg)	2	3
Folic acid (micro gm)	200	2000
Niacin (mg)	15	25--30
Pyridoxine (B6) (mg)	2	20--25
Riboflavin (B 2) (mg)	1.4	2--2.5
Thiamin (B1) (mg)	1.2	9.2
Minerals		
Boron (mg)	N/A	
Calcium (mg)	800	700--1200
Chromium (micro gm)	50-200	300
Copper (mg)	1.5-3	1.5-4
Iodine (micro gm)	150	150
Iron (mg)	10	20
Magnesium (mg)	350	550--600
Manganese (mg)	2-5	10
Phosphorous (mg)	800	800
Potassium (mg)	99	200-500
Selenium (micro gm)	70	200--250
Sodium (mg)	500	400
Zinc (mg)	15	17--20

OXIDATIVE STRESS

When the body reacts with oxygen to produce energy, highly reactive molecules are produced known as free radicals. These interact with other molecules within the cell, which can cause oxidative damage to proteins. Oxidative stress cell damage is induced by reactive oxygen species (ROS) resulting from either an increase in ROS, a decrease ROS protection, or a failure to repair oxidative damage There is a consensus of belief that oxidative damage is related to degenerative diseases such as cancer, Alzheimer's disease, Parkinson's disease, stroke, diabetes, macular degeneration, cataracts, colitis, and irritable bowel syndrome. The degradation by oxidation is the most comprehensive theory of ageing**.** The main damage to cells results from the oxidation of macromolecules such as polyunsaturated fatty acids in membrane lipids, essential proteins, and DNA. High blood sugar from consumption of excess carbohydrates and manufactured high fructose corn syrup (HFCS) promotes oxidation of tissues in the body via non-enzymatic reaction called the Maillard reaction.

Maillard reaction: The first scientific account of non-enzymatic reactions involving the browning of sugar was published by the French biochemist Louis Camille Maillard in 1912. He reported that aqueous solutions of amino acids and glucose, or sugar, turned progressively yellow-brown when heated or stored under physiological conditions. This phenomenon, called protein glycation, involves the reaction of a sugar, such as glucose or fructose, with the amino group of proteins. While Maillard's prediction that this reaction occurs in the human body, particularly in diabetic patients, it went unnoticed for the next 50 years. The Maillard reaction became of major interest to researchers in food science and technology. In contrast to the steady progress in understanding the chemistry and significance of the Maillard reaction in food technology, the potential harmful effects of the Maillard reaction in biological systems were largely overlooked until the discovery in 1971 by Trivelli in Italy of non-enzymatically glycated hemoglobin in diabetic patients. Glycation of proteins has been linked to a growing number of diseases and conditions, such as diabetes, cataract, and aging. Sugar can react with proteins in the body in a process called protein glycation. Oxidants can further chemically modify these glycated proteins, producing advanced glycation end products (AGE). The mechanism of formation, accumulation, and tissue toxicity of AGE has emerged as one of the most coherent explanations for the development of many of the pathological complications of diabetes, cancer, and aging. This risk becomes especially relevant in tissues with a slow rate of regeneration, such as the brain, blood vessels, and the heart.

Acrylamide: This chemical forms in certain foods when a natural amino acid called asparagine reacts with certain naturally occurring sugars, such as glucose and fructose, during processing or cooking at high temperatures. Acrylamide is known to cause cancer in animals. The main offenders are deep fried foods such as potato chips and French fries. The Joint FAO/WHO Expert Committee on Food Additives and Contaminants has recently determined that the estimated intake of acrylamide from certain foods may be a human health concern**.** Consumers can lower exposure to acrylamide by avoiding consumption of deep fried high glycemic load food like fries and chips.

Fructose: The introduction of high fructose corn syrup (HFCS) as a substitute sweetener for sucrose in the mid-1970s has contributed to a general increase in fructose consumption in the U.S. diet. A single 12-ounce can of soda has as much as 13 teaspoons of sugar in the form of high fructose corn syrup (HFCS). In addition, since 1970 the amount of soda we drink has more than doubled to about 56 gallons per person a year. In 2001, we consumed 153 pounds of sugar. Sixty-three pounds of it is fructose, according to the U.S. Department of Agriculture. Fructose is passively absorbed. Insulin is used to move glucose to the tissues by facultative diffusion. Fructose does not significantly stimulate insulin production and does not lead to a high-level rise in blood glucose following consumption. Fructose is metabolized to synthesize fatty acids (triglycerides) in the liver. The livers of the rats on the high fructose diet looked like the livers of alcoholics. Researchers at the University of Michigan found that men who consume very high levels of fructose elevated their triglyceride level by 32 percent. As triglyceride enters our blood stream, it makes our cells resistant to insulin. Recent data shows that large amounts of fructose cause insulin resistance, impaired glucose tolerance, elevated triglycerides, increased hunger, and high blood pressure. Iron, magnesium, copper, calcium, and zinc balances tended to be more negative when consuming large amounts of fructose. There is also an increase in uric acid, which causes gout.

Check the list of ingredients in the foods you buy. From an evolutionary standpoint, our bodies cannot handle large quantities of carbohydrates and sugars (particularly HFCS). Eating it poses a health hazard!

Antioxidants: Free radicals are atoms or groups of atoms with an odd (unpaired) number of electrons and can be formed when oxygen interacts with certain molecules. Once formed these highly reactive radicals can start a chain reaction. Their chief danger comes from the damage they can do when they react with cellular components. Cells may function poorly, die, or advanced glycation products (AGE) may formed by the oxidation of glucose and proteins. An AGE is a cancer promoting substance. To prevent free radical damage the body has a defense system of antioxidants. Antioxidants are intimately involved in the prevention of cellular damage, which is the common pathway for cancer, aging, and a variety of diseases. Antioxidants are chemical substances that donate an electron to the free radical and convert it to a harmless molecule. Antioxidants intercept free radicals and protect cells from the oxidative damage that leads to aging and disease. Antioxidants prevent injury to blood vessel membranes, helping to optimize blood flow to the heart and brain, defend against cancer-causing DNA damage, and help lower the risk of cardiovascular disease and dementia. Some antioxidants are made in our cells and include glutathione, coenzyme *Q-10* and lipoic acid. Other essential antioxidants such as vitamin *C, E*, and selenium must be obtained from our diet. Antioxidants abound in vitamins, minerals, and botanicals. Here is a list of some of the major antioxidants:

1. Alpha-Lipolic Acid synergistically works with vitamin C, E, and Glutathione.
2. Bioflavonoids include many plant compounds such as procyanidolic oligomers (pycnogenols) in pine bark and grape seed, Bilberry herb, Rutin from citrus fruits, Hesperidin from citrus fruits, Quercetin from apple and onions, and Cucurmin in turmeric spice, Ginkgo biloba herb, epigallocatechin-gallate (EGCG) in green tea, and Carotenoids. Colors indicate type. Alpha carotene is orange in carrots, lutein is the green in spinach, lycopene is red in tomatoes.
3. CoQ10 (Ubiquinone) is a primary antioxidant made by the body also found in fish, beef, peanuts, and spinach.
4. Glutathione is the cell's primary antioxidant made by the body. Take 100 mg of Alpha lipoic acid to increase production.
5. Selenium is a trace mineral needed for formation of Glutathione.

6. Vitamin E tocopherol is a fat-soluble vitamin that has several forms. Vitamin E can be found in nuts, seeds, vegetable and fish oils, whole grains (esp. wheat germ), fortified cereals, and apricots. See current ODA in the vitamins table.
7. Vitamin C, ascorbic acid, is a water-soluble vitamin present in citrus fruits and juices, green peppers, cabbage, spinach, broccoli, kale, cantaloupe, kiwi, and strawberries.
8. Beta-carotene is a precursor (converted by the body) to vitamin A (retinol) and is present in liver, egg yolk, milk, butter, spinach, carrots, squash, broccoli, yams, tomato, cantaloupe, peaches, and grains. Vitamin A has no antioxidant properties and can be toxic when taken in excess.
9. Cysteine is the amino acid precursor to Glutathione. Supplemental form is L-Cysteine.
10. Melatonin is a hormone produced by pineal gland implicated in sleep patterns and has antioxidant properties.
11. Superoxide Dismutase (SOD) is made by the body and is bound to copper/zinc or manganese. SOD decreased with age but is available as supplement. The substrate binding metals must be available.
12. Zinc: Trace metal necessary for several antioxidant related compounds.

Epidemiologic observations show lower cancer rates in people whose diets are rich in fruits and vegetables. Thus far, none of the large, well-designed studies has shown that supplementation with antioxidants reduces the risk of cancer. Antioxidants are also thought to have a role in slowing the aging process and preventing heart disease and strokes, but the data is still inconclusive. Perhaps the best advice is to eat fruit and vegetables in abundance.

These are the USDA top 20 Antioxidant Foods.

1. Small red beans (dried)	11. Strawberries
2. Wild blueberries	12. Red Delicious apples
3. Red kidney beans	13. Granny Smith apples
4. Pinto beans	14. Pecans
5. Blueberries (cultivated)	15. Sweet cherries
6. Cranberries	16. Black plums
7. Artichokes (cooked)	17. Russet potatoes (cooked)
8. Blackberries	18. Black beans (dried)
9. Prunes	19. Plums
10. Raspberries	20. Gala apples

A major barrier is a lack of consensus on uniform antioxidant measurements. A study from Tufts University in Boston ranks the antioxidant value using a test tube analysis that measures the total antioxidant power of foods called Oxygen Radical Absorbance Capacity (ORAC).

Top-scoring fruits and vegetables ORAC (3½ ounces)

Fruits:	**Vegetables:**
Prunes -- 5570	Kale -- 11770
Raisins – 2830 (also high glycemic load)	Spinach -- 11260
Blueberries -- 2400	Brussels sprout -- 1980
Blackberries -- 2036	Alfalfa sprouts -- 1930
Strawberries -- 1540	Broccoli Flowers -- 1890
Raspberries -- 1220	Beets -- 1840
Plums -- 949	Red bell pepper -- 1710
Oranges -- 750	Onion -- 1450
Red grapes -- 739	Corn -- 1400
Cherries -- 670	Eggplant -- 1390
Kiwi fruit -- 602	
Grapefruit, pink -- 483	

Some antioxidants tend to recycle and refresh each other. Dr Lester Packer, in his book, *The Antioxidant Miracle*, suggests including these recycled antioxidants.

Recycled Antioxidants

Antioxidant	**Daily dose**
Lipoic Acid(ALA)	100 mg-recycles all
Vitamin E	200 mg d-alpha, 200 mg mixed tocopherols, 100 mg tocotrienols
Vitamin C	1000mg slow release +rose hips
CoQ10	30 mg
Glutathione	increased by lipoic acid
Flavonoids	Ginkgo biloba 30 mg
Carotenoids	0 mg (3 orange fruits, 2 green leafy vegs)
Selenium	200-250 mcg

Phytochemicals: Phytochemicals are non-nutritive plant chemicals that have protective or disease preventive properties. There are more than a thousand known phytochemicals. It is well known that plants produce these chemicals for protection. Recent research demonstrates that many phytochemicals can protect humans against diseases. Some of the well-known phytochemicals are lycopene in tomatoes, isoflavones in soy and flavanoids in fruits. Phytochemicals are not essential nutrients and are not required by the human body for sustaining life.

There are many phytochemicals and each works differently:

1. Antioxidant - Most phytochemicals have antioxidant activity, which protects cells against oxidative damage. Some have been listed in previous section.
2. Hormonal action - Isoflavones, found in soy, imitate human estrogens and help to reduce menopausal symptoms and osteoporosis.
3. Stimulation of enzymes - Indoles, the phytochemical found in cabbages, stimulate enzymes that make the estrogen less effective and could reduce the risk for breast cancer. Other phytochemicals, which interfere with enzymes, are protease inhibitors (soy and beans), terpenes (citrus fruits and cherries).
4. Interference with DNA replication - Saponins found in beans interferes with the replication of cell DNA, thereby preventing the multiplication of cancer cells. Capsaicin, found in hot peppers, protects DNA from carcinogens.
5. Anti-bacterial effect - The phytochemical allicin from garlic has anti-bacterial properties.

Phytochemicals are found in most fruit and vegetable foods. The color pigments are an indication of the existence of phytochemicals. The table below lists the phytochemical family and examples of foods that contain them.

Phytochemicals and their Food Sources

Phytochemical Family:	Food Sources
Ally Sulfides	Onions, garlic, leeks, chives
Indoles	Broccoli, cabbage, kale
Isoflavones	Soybeans
Isothiocyanates	Cruciferous vegetables
Phenolic acids	Tomatoes, citrus fruits, carrots,
Ellagic & ferulic acid	Green tea, grapes, wine
Saponins	Beans and legumes
Terpenes	Cherries, citrus fruit peel

Resveratrol: This remarkable antioxidant was first isolated from the roots of the Ko-jo-kon plant and subsequently discovered as the active antioxidant in red wine. Resveratrol has been shown to be active in the inhibition of radical oxygen products, inhibition of lipid per oxidation, down-regulation of proinflammatory mediators, and cancer chemotherapeutic effects. All good stuff. The food wheel allows one to two glasses of red wine daily.

There is widespread scientific agreement that eating adequate amounts of fruits and vegetables can help lower the incidence of cardiovascular disease and certain cancers. With respect to antioxidants and other phytochemicals, the key question is whether supplementation has been proven to do more good than harm. So far, the answer is not in evidence, which is why the FDA will not permit any of these substances to be labeled or marketed with claims that they can prevent disease.

There is a growing body of evidence that supports the importance of antioxidants and supplements. The Food Wheel recommends considering a daily multivitamin plus minerals. Consider supplementation with recycled antioxidants. May add one to two glasses of red wine.

ARTIFICIAL SWEETENERS

Aspartame: Aspartame is aspartic acid and phenylalanine held in chemical bond by Methanol. Aspartame is 10% Methanol by weight and breaks down into Formic acid (the venom in ant stings), Formaldehyde (embalming fluid), and Diketopiperazine (the brain tumor agent). Labels for both prescription and nonprescription products must include the phenylalanine content. Headaches are the most common adverse side effect attributed to aspartame. Up to 11% of patients with chronic migraine, headaches reported headaches triggered by aspartame. Aspartame has been linked to various neuropsychiatric disorders, including panic attacks, mood changes, visual hallucinations, manic episodes, and isolated dizziness. A small, double-blind crossover study of patients with major depression revealed a higher incidence of reactions in these patients compared with nondepressed volunteers after administration of 30 mg/kg for 7 days. Symptoms included headache, nervousness, dizziness, memory impairment, nausea, temper outbursts, and depression. Seizures have been reported via passive surveillance data collected by the FDA and in a few case reports. The methanol toxicity mimics multiple sclerosis.

In spite off all of the preceding, none of these conditions has been rigorously proven to be caused by aspartame.

Saccharin: Foods containing saccharin no longer carry a label stating that the "use of this product may be hazardous to your health ...contains saccharin which has been determined to cause cancer in laboratory animals." The American FDA lifted this warning in 2001, as saccharin no longer has been connected to cancer in human beings. Many remain skeptical.

Sucralose: Sucralose, sold as Splenda, is a chlorinated sucrose derivative. Pre-approval research showed that sucralose caused shrunken thymus glands (up to 40% shrinkage) and enlarged liver and kidneys. The manufacturer claims that the chlorine added to sucralose is similar to the chlorine atom in the salt (NaCl) molecule. Sucralose may be more like ingesting tiny amounts of chlorinated pesticides. We will never know without long-term, independent human research or decades of use. Not withstanding, it is the best commercially available yet.

Stevia: Another sweetener, stevioside, is championed by natural-foods advocates in the United States and is used in several countries. Stevioside comes from the leaves of the stevia plant (Stevia rebaudiana Bertoni). It is stable to 200°C (392°F), but it is not fermentable and does not act in browning reactions (see Maillard reaction).In the 1970s, the Japanese government approved the plant for use in food. FDA considers stevia leaves and stevioside as unapproved, non- Generally Recognized as Safe [GRAS] food additives. In 1992, the American Herbal Products Association (AHPA) petitioned the FDA to declare stevia as GRAS. The FDA rejected AHPA's petition, contending inadequate evidence to approve the product. The agency does allow the herb to be used in dietary supplements as covered by DSHEA (Dietary Supplement Health and Education Act).

Tagatose: Naturlose is the brand name for tagatose. It looks like sugar, tastes like sugar, cooks like sugar. Technically, it is sugar. However, it is sugar with almost no calories. It is 100-percent natural, not synthesized or derived from sugar. Scientifically known as D-tagatose, Tagatose occurs naturally in some dairy products and other foods. The patented production process starts from whey. Tagatose has been determined to be a Generally Recognized as Safe (GRAS) substance in the U.S. Tagatose has also been determined GRAS for use in cosmetics and toothpastes, as well as in drugs. The chemical formulas for fructose and tagatose are identical. The two molecules look the same, but in tagatose, one atom of carbon juts off to the left (Levo-sugar) of the main structure instead of off to right (Dextro-sugar) as it does in fructose. It is a confusing chemical to the human body. To the tongue, it tastes just like regular sugar. However, the body has never swallowed left- handed sugar and cannot digest it. Diabetics can eat foods sweetened with tagatose without changes in their blood glucose levels. Unfortunately, Naturlose is not readily available in stores.

Sugar alcohols: Sugar alcohols also known as polyols, are a common ingredient in many processed foods. They are found naturally in berries, apples, plums and are produced commercially from carbohydrates. They contain about 1/2 the carbohydrate in an equal amount of table sugar and require little or no insulin. When eaten to excess (20-50 grams) alcohol sugars can cause abdominal discomfort, bloating, and a laxative effect.

Sorbitol is the alcohol form of sucrose. It occurs naturally in fruits and vegetables. It is manufactured from corn syrup. Sorbitol has been used for many years in the diet, especially of diabetics. There have been no indications of significant harmful effects.

Xylitol, also called "wood sugar," is the alcohol form of xylose. It occurs naturally in straw, corncobs, fruit, vegetables, and some seaweed. For use in food manufacturing, xylitol is extracted from birch wood chips. Xylitol is used as a sweetener in chewing gums and other dietetic products.

Mannitol is the alcohol form of mannose. It occurs naturally in pineapples, olives, asparagus, sweet potatoes, and carrots. Mannitol is extracted from seaweed for use in food manufacturing. It is sometimes used as a sweetener in dietetic products.

Maltitol is about 0.9 times as sweet as sucrose. It is a disaccharide polyol produced by the hydrogenation of maltose. It occurs widely in nature (e.g., in chicory and roasted malt).

Less well-known sugar alcohols include Galactitol, Erythritol, Inositol, Ribitol, Dithioerythritol, Dithiothreitol, and Glycerol.

About half our sugar consumption comes from invisible sugars in processed foods. The Food Wheel advises utilization of sugar substitutes such as Splenda or Naturlose.

FOOD ADDITIVES

Food Additives are substances added to foods by manufacturers ostensibly to prevent spoilage or to improve appearance, taste, texture, or nutritive value. Food additives comprise about 10% of the food consumed by the average adult. The average person consumes more than four pounds of additives each year. There are now approximately 3000 approved additives. As nutritional awareness grows, many health experts and consumers have become more vocal in their criticism of the excessive and potentially dangerous use of food additives. Others point to a conspiracy where additives are used synergistically to stimulate consumer appetite.

Food additives serve five main roles:

Maintain product consistency. Emulsifiers provide a consistent texture and prevent products from separating. Stabilizers and thickeners provide a uniform texture. Anticaking agents enable substances to flow freely.

Improve or preserve the nutrient value. Fortification and enrichment of foods has made it possible to improve the nutritional status of population. For example, vitamins and minerals are added to many foods including flour, cereal, margarine, and milk. This helps to make up for vitamins or minerals that may be low or lacking in an individual's diet.

Maintain the wholesomeness and the palatability of foods. Contamination from bacteria can allow food-borne illnesses to occur. Preservatives reduce the spoilage that air, fungi, bacteria, or yeast can cause. Preservatives such as antioxidants help baked goods preserve their flavor by preventing the fats and oils from becoming rancid. They also keep fresh fruits from turning brown when exposed to air.

Control the acidity and alkalinity, and to provide leavening. Specific additives aid to adjustment of the acidity or alkalinity of foods to gain a wished taste, color, or flavor. Leavening agents that release acids when they are heated react with baking soda to help biscuits, cakes, and other baked goods rise.

Provide color and improve flavor. Certain colors improve appearance of foods. Many spices, natural extracts, and synthetic flavors bring out the best in the flavor of food.

Shopping was easy when most food came from farms. Now, factory-made foods have made chemical additives a significant part of our diet. Unless you already buy all organic and natural foods, over 90% of the food produced today contain hydrogenated or partially hydrogenated oil. If you are eating more chicken, turkey, and fish, because it is healthier, you may be surprised to learn that sliced chicken and turkey from the deli contains nitrites. Nitrites, a preservative, are found in almost all processed meats, including luncheon meats, hot dogs, sausages, and bacon. Then there is tuna, a healthy choice if it only contains tuna and water. However, most tuna contains broth or vegetable protein, which contains MSG. The catch is that additives are not required to be listed on the label if it is an ingredient in the broth, not directly added to the product. This is the way food manufacturers hide MSG in the food they produce. In addition, hidden MSG can be a very serious problem to those who are sensitive to it. MSG can cause a wide variety of symptoms including migraines, numbness and tingling, asthma, seizures, diarrhea, panic attacks and heart problems. Other sources of hidden MSG include autolyzed yeast, bouillon, stock, malt extract, malt flavoring, barley malt, maltodextrin, natural flavors, pectin, seasonings, carrageenan, soy sauce, soy protein, whey protein, anything enzyme modified, fermented, protein fortified, or ultrapasteurized, fast foods, chips, condiments, salad dressings, lunch meats, sausages and soups. In fact, most processed foods contain MSG.

What does the 5% labeling loophole say? If the amount of an ingredient in a food is less than 5% of the food (such as 4.5 per cent sunflower oil added to soymilk), a food additive (such as antioxidant TBHQ, 319) in that ingredient does not have to be included in the ingredients list on the label unless the food additive is performing a technological function in the final food. Who decides is the additive is performing a technological function? The food manufacturers decide. Consumption of the unlisted food additive could effect consumers. Here are some additives to avoid:

- MSG and Free Glutamates
- Artificial colorings
- Propyl gallate
- Acacia gum, Alginic acid, and Benzoic acid
- Iron salt
- Nitrites and Nitrate
- BHA and BHT
- Brominated vegetable oil (BVO)
- Olestra or Olean
- Sulfites
- High fructose corn syrup (HFCS)

These are used primarily in foods of low nutritional value. One popular food example is the Twinkie. The ingredients are wheat flour, ferrous sulphate, niacin, thiamine, riboflavin, folic acid, sugar, high fructose corn syrup, vegetable and animal shortening, dextrose, whole eggs, and twenty other ingredients not specified. Do not forget the two most familiar food additives, sugar, and salt. They may pose the greatest risk because we consume so much.

Food Wheel states that processed foods will include additives, which are detrimental to your long-term health. Avoid excessive use of products in bag, box, or can. Read the food label. If you read the ingredients and you do not know what it is and cannot pronounce it, maybe you should not consume in excess, or not at all.

FOOD LABEL BASICS

The food label is the only information mandated by law. Other statements on the package are advertisement, not health information. Here is a rundown of the basics you will find on a food label and how you can use the information to improve your daily diet: **Remember- processed foods contain added salt, fat, and sugar**

Nutrition Facts ● 1
Serving Size 1 cup (253g) ● 2
Servings Per Container 4

Amount Per Serving	
Calories 260	Calories from Fat 70 ● 3
● 4	**% Daily Value***
Total Fat 8g ● 5	**13%**
Saturated Fat 3g	**17%**
Cholesterol 130mg ● 6	**44%**
Sodium 1010mg	**42%**
Total Carbohydrate 22g ● 7	**7%**
Dietary Fiber 9g	**36%**
Sugars 4g	
Protein 25g ● 8	
Vitamin A 35% ●	Vitamin C 2%
Calcium 6% ●● 9	Iron 30%

*Percent Daily Values are based on a 2,000 calorie diet. Your daily values may be higher or lower depending on your calorie needs: ● 10

		Calories: 2000	2,500
Total Fat	Less than	65g	80g
Sat Fat	Less than	20g	25g
Cholesterol	Less than	300mg	300mg
Sodium	Less than	2,400mg	2,400mg
Total Carbohydrate		300g	375g
Dietary Fiber		25g	30g

Calories per gram: ● 11
Fat 9 • Carbohydrate 4 • Protein 4

1. Title: When you see the title "Nutrition Facts," you know this is the current information label approved by the Food and Drug Administration.

2. Serving Sizes: Serving sizes are standardized, so you can compare similar products with one another. The serving sizes on the label are **supposed** to be close to "real life" serving size. The information on the rest of the label is based on data for one serving. Remember, a package may contain more than one serving. That is what the **servings per container** line tell you.

Energy Density for one serving is 260cal/253g=1.03

3. Calories from Fat: The closer this number is to the food's total calories, the fatter the food contains. Try to find foods with lowest amounts of calories from fat.

4. Daily Value %: This information is based on a 2,000-calorie daily diet. You may need more or less. **Your weight x 12 = calories you are eating now.** Reduce your calories by 500-1000 per day.

5. Fat: Total fat is important to watch, but saturated fat is particularly bad for you. Saturated fat raises your blood cholesterol level and that could lead to heart troubles. On new labels Trans fat must now appear along with total fat, saturated fat, and cholesterol **Otherwise, you have to read the contents.**

6. Cholesterol, Sodium: Along with the saturated-fat information above, cholesterol amounts are important for anyone concerned about heart disease. High levels of cholesterol can lead to serious heart problems later in life. Sodium (or salt) levels are important to monitor if you have high-blood pressure. [Keep less than 2000mg sodium/day]

7. Carbohydrates: These fit into two categories dietary fiber and carbohydrates (sugars). You want to eat more fiber and fewer simple carbohydrates.

8. Protein: The food label does not specify a daily percentage or guideline for protein consumption because so much depends on individual needs. An athlete needs more than an office worker does, but in a typical 2,000-calorie diet, most people need no more than 50 grams of protein per day.

9. Vitamins and Minerals: The FDA requires only Vitamin A, Vitamin C, Iron, and Calcium on this label, although food companies can voluntarily list others. The FDA feels these four vitamins and minerals are particularly important in order to maintain a healthy diet.

10. Daily Values Footnote: The daily values footnote is a reminder of how many calories are in each gram of fat, carbohydrate, and protein.

11. Calories per Gram Footnote: Shows the calories for each macronutrient.

As mandated by the Nutrition Labeling and Education Act of 1990, the Food and Drug Administration has issued final food labeling rules for health claims. The rules, published in the Jan. 6, 1993, Federal Register, allow claims about seven relationships:

- Calcium and a reduced risk of osteoporosis (a condition of lowered bone mass).
- Sodium and an increased risk of hypertension (high blood pressure).
- Dietary saturated fat and cholesterol and an increased risk of coronary heart disease.
- Dietary fat and an increased risk of cancer.
- Fiber-containing grain products, fruits, and vegetables and a reduced risk of cancer.
- Fruits, vegetables, and grain products that contain fiber, particularly soluble fiber, and a reduced risk of coronary heart disease.
- Fruits, vegetables, and a reduced risk of cancer.

Eight major foods: milk, eggs, fish, shellfish, nuts and peanuts, wheat, and soybeans account for 90 percent of all documented food allergic reactions. In 2004, Congress passed a law requiring food manufacturers to label any ingredients derived from these eight allergens in clear language.

Refer back to your food wheel and you will see that by eating non-processed foods such as vegetables, fruits, fish, whole grains, and low fat dairy; you will avoid eating extra fat, salt, and sugar.

MEASUREMENTS, SERVINGS AND PORTIONS

Processed food manufacturers are a source of confusion with regard to serving size. They print numbers on the package based on an unrealistically small serving. Look at the "Servings per container" line along with the calories. A can of Cream of Mushroom soup contains 100 calories per serving. A serving size is 4 oz. There are two and three quarter's servings per can! You might assume the whole can of soup was 100 calories. By reading the fine print you see that each can of soup actually adds up to 275 calories. The 100 calories is for 8 tablespoons without water! In addition, potato chip serving is one ounce. No one ever eats an ounce of potato chips either. A serving is 150 calories for one ounce. That is about 1200 calories for an 8-ounce bag. That is enough calories for a person to maintain body functions at rest for a day. Note that soup is fluid oz and potato chip is weight oz. Here are serving sizes listed according to food groups.

1. Fruit and Vegetable Groups: One fruit and vegetable serving is equal to one piece the size of a tennis ball or 1/2 cup the size of a light bulb.
2. Cereals, Rice, Pasta, and other Grains Group: 1 slice bread or 1/2 bagel the size of a hockey puck. 1/2 cup of cooked rice equals a cupcake wrapper. 1/2 cup pasta equals an ice cream scoop.
3. Meat, Chicken, Fish, Dry Beans and Peas, Eggs, and Nuts Group: Three ounces lean meat, chicken, or fish measures up to a deck of cards or a checkbook.
4. Dairy Group: One-ounce cheese equals about the size of four dice.
5. Fats, Oils, and Sweets Group: A teaspoon of fat looks like the tip of your thumb.

Conversions-liquid

Pinch or dash = less than 1/8 teaspoon
3 teaspoons = 1 tablespoon
2 tablespoons = 1 fluid oz.
4 tablespoons = 1/4 cup = 2 ounces
6 tablespoons = 3/4 cup
5 1/8 tablespoons = 1/3 cup
8 tablespoons = 1/2 cup
16 tablespoons = 1 cup
1 cup = 8 fluid oz.
2 cups = 1 pint
4 cups = 2 pints = 1 quart
4 quarts = 1 gallon
2 cups liquid = 16 oz. = 1 pound

Conversion-Weight

1 lb	453.6 g
lb	0.4536kg
oz	28.35g
kg	2.2046lb
kg	1,000,000mg
kg	1,000g
g	1,000
g	1,000,000µg
mg	1,000ug

Note that fluid oz is not equal to oz weight
You can convert online at http://www.onlineconversion.com/

READINESS FOR CHANGE

Often there is a lack confidence in our ability to make changes successfully. The pros and cons need to be listed. Set goals in small achievable steps. List the barriers to change and have a plan to overcome them. Recognizing barriers and achieving lasting change may require the help of professional counseling.

The five stages of motivational readiness can be applied to dieting, exercise, or life changes. The contemplative statements to oneself reflect the stage of readiness for change:

1. Stage One: **Precontemplation**. I have no intention of changing.
2. Stage Two: **Contemplation**. I intend to change at some future time.
3. Stage Three: **Preparation**. I am ready to change within the next month.
4. Stage Four: **Action**. I have recently changed a behavior.
5. Stage Five: **Maintenance**. I have carried out the new behavior for at least six months to two years.

It is imperative that your relationship with food is changed:

1. **Make small changes that fit in with your life.** Set your goal to small measurable changes. Chose from the Food Wheel rules.
2. **Make sure that you are eating enough to avoid feeling hungry.** You are more likely to eat more when you are hungry. Good tip to avoid hunger is to choose fresh fruits and vegetables for snacks.

3. **Make long-term lifestyle changes.** Keeping your weight under control is not about whether you have willpower. It is more important you be committed to long-term lifestyle changes like Food Wheel choices and daily exercise. Realistic changes can become part of your every day life.
4. **Plan room for restraint.** Rather than creating hard and fast rules about your diet, practice restraint. Make healthy choices most of the time. People who practice restraint do not feel they have lapsed. They are able to return to their Food Wheel plan.
5. **Work out why you eat more than you need.** If your eating is due to an emotional need, you may benefit from counseling. What moods trigger your appetite? Are your eating habits linked to certain situations or times of the day? You can also work out alternative ways to reward and comfort yourself. If you choose appropriate Food Wheel items, you can substitute previous energy dense foods.
6. **Learn new habits.** There is an old saying: "Old behaviors will not produce new results." Make sensible changes to your lifestyle.
7. **Controlling your eating is only half the battle.** Healthy Food Wheel eating is only one part of the equation. The other key factor is exercise and activity.
8. **Start a food inventory.** Write down everything you eat for three -five days. List in columns for each food group. Then convert the amounts to calories using one of the popular calorie count books like *Harriet Roth's Fat Counter* [$3.99]. This will give you an idea of the total calories you are eating and in which category. Refer to the Food Wheel groups: carbohydrate, fat, and protein. Note how much white carbohydrates, solid fats, dairy, and non-lean meats you consume. This would be a good first goal to change the types of

foods you eat. Reduce total calories by 500/day. You will be able to do this by changing to fruits, vegetables, lean meats and fish, and avoiding white carbohydrates. Incorporate a food log in your food diary. Look for opportunities to change eating habits.

9. **Keep a food diary.** Keep a diary of your weekly weight and a daily narrative of what you ate and problems you are having. Start with one or two of the Food Wheel Rules. You must write your goals, celebrate your successes, and note your setbacks.

example food inventory one day						
Food	**carb**	**fat**	**fruit**	**veg**	**protein**	**dairy**
apple			81			
Orange juice 2 cup			112			
milk whole						149
Cheerios-2 cups	250					
Pizza sub	464					
Beer can	146					
Chicken breast					200	
Pizza-2 slices	510			150		
TOTAL=2062 calories	1370		193	150	200	149

Appropriate action:	**Calories saved**
1. Reduce carbohydrates (pizza).	-510
2. Increase vegetables.	+50
3. Change to skim milk	-49
4. Reduce orange juice to one cup.	-56
5. Avoid cold cereals (cheerios) use fruit.	-170

A Savings of 735 calories is more than a pound a week!

Food Wheel Rules

- Drink eight glasses of water every day.
- Daily, exercise to your capacity.
- For weight maintenance calories = weight x 12.
- Reduce daily intake by 500 calories if BMI >25.
- Fresh fruits and vegetables any time.
- Limit sodium to 2000 mg a day.
- Limit sweet drinks and juice. Avoid high fructose corn syrup (HFCS).
- Avoid white carbohydrates, GL >10.
- Avoid fats that are solid. Use Canola oil or fish oil high in omega 3.
- Foods in a bag, box, or can have extra salt, sugar, or fat.
- Eat vegetables raw anytime. Not potatoes or yams.
- Choose only one dairy/hormone/lactase product a day.
- May consume one or two glasses of red wine daily.
- Multivitamins with minerals for most over 50 years old.
- Choose lean meats such as poultry and fish.
- Choose foods with energy density (ED) of 2 or less.
- Advertised high fiber foods contain considerable carbohydrates, salt, and fat.
- Use the Food wheel to guide food purchase.
- Read the USDA food labels, the rest is advertisement, not health information.
- Every thing you buy you will eventually eat.
- Extra energy consumed is extra energy conserved

Additional Helpful Dieting Hints:

1. Avoid alcohol before meals when dieting. This could disinhibit you and allow you to eat more.
2. Add inulin based fiber tablets before meals.
3. Eat five small Food Wheel meals each day instead of one or two large ones.
4. Don't skip meals. This leads to over eating later in the day.
5. Place a copy of the Food Wheel on your refrigerator.
6. Eat very S-L-O-W-L-Y with the first 5 bites in 20 minutes
7. Do not ever skip breakfast.
8. Eat nothing after 8:00pm
9. Snack on fruits and vegetables or unsweetened drink.
10. Drink a glass of water, or unsweetened tea before meals.
11. Downsize the plate you eat from to reduce your portion.
12. Keep an eating diary.
13. Use sugar substitutes such as Splenda.

THERE IS NO MAGIC PILL

Diet pills target several areas:

1. Burn more calories by speeding up your metabolism.
2. Block the utilization of carbohydrates in your gut.
3. Include substances that suppress appetite.
4. Bind with fat in your gut to retard digestion.

Diet pills are either FDA prescription drugs or over the counter (OTC) Supplements. There are only a few prescription weight loss medicines but hundreds of OTC supplements.

Xenical: Approved by the FDA in 1999, is a new class of anti-obesity drugs known as lipase inhibitors. Xenical decreases dietary fat absorption by 30 percent. Undigested fats are not absorbed so fewer calories are available to the body. The main side effects of Xenical are cramping, diarrhea, flatulence, intestinal discomfort, and leakage of oily stool.

Meridia (sibutramine): approved by the FDA in 1997 is classed as a selective serotonin reuptake inhibitor (SSRI). Serotonin is responsible for mood, appetite, nausea, sexuality, and sleep. Other SSRI drugs are used for treatment of depression and anxiety. One drug in the same class, Prozac, has been used for weight loss. St John's wort is an OTC herb that is used to treat depression and is included in many diet products. Treating depression should always be considered because depression can be a major component of overeating. It should be noted that there is also a general side effect of weight gain with the SSRI class of antidepressants. This may be attributed to the fact that these drugs block serotonin degradation in the brain but do not add serotonin to the system. People with uncontrolled high blood pressure, heart disease, congestive heart failure, irregular heartbeat, or stroke should not use Meridia. Side effects of Meridia include headache, dry mouth, constipation, and insomnia. Meridia, unlike other SSRI drugs, is a controlled substance.

Other Prescription drugs: Anti-obesity prescription drugs such as Bontril (phendimetrazine tartrate), Desoxyn (methamphetamine) and Ionamin and Adipex-P (phentermine) were approved by the FDA many years ago. They are "speed" drugs that should not be used by people with heart disease, high blood pressure, an overactive thyroid gland, or glaucoma. These drugs are approved only for short-term use and have significant potential for physical dependence or addiction.

OTC Diet supplements: Billions of dollars of diet products and services sold each year. Dietary Supplement Health and Education Act (1994) states that a dietary supplement is a product (not tobacco) that is intended to supplement the diet. Contains one or more dietary ingredients (including vitamins, minerals, herbs or other botanicals, amino acids, and other substances). Is intended to be taken by mouth as a pill, capsule, tablet, or liquid. Is labeled on the front panel as being a dietary supplement. Complete information is available at the National Institute of Health website: http://ods.od.nih.gov/factsheets/DietarySupplements.asp.

Brain food: Increasing the levels of serotonin in the brain tends to suppress appetite. 5-HTP is the precursor chemical to serotonin and there is some evidence that supports appetite suppression and increased mood. The serotonin molecule will not pass from to the blood into the brain because it is too large. Therefore, the precursors 5-HTP and tryptophan can increase the conversion to serotonin in the brain. L-tyrosine supplementation increases brain norepinphrine levels. Vitamin B6, or pyridoxine, is the cofactor for enzymes that facilitates conversion. Excessive B6 may cause conversion in the liver, which bypasses the brain. Other vitamins and minerals connected to brain health are E, B1, B12, magnesium, and Folic acid. There are OTC products that contain herbs, vitamins, and minerals, which are advertised as supplementation to brain chemicals and provide gains in memory, energy, and weight loss. Supplementation with 5-HTP or an OTC complex may be helpful or just decrease the size of your wallet instead of your waste. Refer back to the ODA vitamin recommendations.

There are several truths about OTC weight loss supplements:

Truth: Advertisements promise unachievable goals.

Truth: The diet industry relies on your failure.

Truth: Venders write most information.

Truth: Few reliable studies show efficacy.

Truth: It is not in the diet supplement industry's economic interest to provide the truth.

The ingredients of supplements can vary widely. There is no one universal magical ingredient. Some products tout one herb or enzyme as "the answer" to weight loss. Usually they contain combinations of, digestive enzymes, herbs, multivitamins, and minerals such as the following:

Acetyl L-Carnitine, Green Tea, Camellia Sinensis, Alpha Lipoic Acid, Bioperine, Piper Nigrum, BiotinCassia Angustifolia, Capsicum Frutescens, Plantago Major, Xanthum Gum, Fucus Vesiculosus, Konjac Radix, Echinacea Purpurea, Ananas Comosus, Allium Sativum, Zingiber Officinale, Panax Ginseng, Llex Paraguariensis, Filipendula Ulmaria, Hypericum Perforatum, Valeriana Officianalis N-Acetyl L-tyrosine, Gymnema sylvestre leaf extract standardized for gymnemic acids, ginger root, Ginkgo biloba leaf extract standardized for ginkgo flavoneglycosides and sesquiterpene lactones, Capsicum fruit, Trimethylglycine hydrochloride, Banaba leaf extract standardized for corosolic acid, Fulvic acid (from shilajit), Bioperine® black pepper extract, and vanadium (35 mcg as vanadium amino acid chelate). Simmondsin Extract, Spirulina velvet Bean standardized for Macuna Pruiens, Citrus aurantium extract, Nut Grass extract standardized for Octopamine, L-Glutamine, 5-HTP, Lecithin standardized for phosphatides, Rhodiola rosea root extract standardized for rosavins, Phosphatidylserine, and Coleus forskohlii tuber extract). Chromium, Phase 2 Brand White Kidney Bean Extract, Hoodia Gordonii, Magnesium, Garcia Cambogia Extract.

There are no large population controlled trials that support the efficacy of any of these substances, alone or in combination, as a weight loss medicine.

Future diet medicine: Recent studies show that adipose tissue (fat cells) is a highly active endocrine organ. Hormones like, ghrelin, leptin, adiponectin, obestatin, and resistin have important roles in energy homeostasis, glucose metabolism, lipid metabolism, reproduction, cardiovascular function, and immunity. Leptin, adiponectin, and resistin are produced by the adipose tissue. The protein leptin is a satiety hormone which regulates appetite and energy balance of the body. Leptin has demonstrated some success in rat models but not in humans. Obese humans seem to exhibit leptin resistance. Increased resistin concentrations might cause insulin resistance and thus could link obesity with type II diabetes. Ghrelin and Obestatin are produced in the stomach and are encoded by the same gene. Both have a role in long-term regulation of energy metabolism and short-term regulation of feeding. Ghrelin and Obestatin have opposite effects of stimulating/suppressed food intake, stimulating/inhibited jejunal (intestine) contraction, and increasing/decreased body-weight. Research concerning the hormonal drivers of appetite stimulation and suppression will provide an approved medicine in a few years.

There are four contenders at present:

1. CYT009-GhrQ vaccine uses the immune system to bind Ghrelin and therefore suppress hunger.
2. Acomplia (rimonabant) is a cannabinoid (marijuana) derivative that suppresses hunger and smoking. French pharmaceutical company Sanofi-Aventis is applying for FDA license to market in USA in 2006.
3. Oxyntomodulin is a hormone found in the intestine which when injected hits receptors in the brain to produce a feeling of fullness.
4. Spiegemler is a drug that binds to Ghrelin directly and suppresses hunger. The German pharmaceutical company Noxxon Pharma has presently found it significant in animal studies.

PARTING WORDS

There are many competing views about what to eat and what not to eat. It is incumbent upon you to question all information regarding nutrition and food choices. Much of the conventional wisdom about what to eat does not have evidence based support. It is usually false advertisement or flawed reporting. The news media and health care professionals can be misinformed and even biased. When you read or hear reports about a study that indicates specific findings in the popular press, rarely are the details of the study given. Read the actual research articles and ask questions. Remember the following critical thinking hints.

1. An association between two events is not the same as a cause and effect.

2. Demonstrating one link in a postulated chain of events does not mean that the whole chain is proved.

3. Probabilities are not the same as certainties.

4. The way a scientific result is framed can greatly affect its impact.

SELECTED REFERENCES

Agus MS, Swain JF, Larson CL, et al. Dietary composition and physiologic adaptations to energy restriction. *Am J Clin Nutr.* 2000; 71:901-907.

Albu J, Konnaaarides C, Pi-Sunyer. FX: Weight control: metabolic and cardiovascular effects. *Diabetes Rev.* 1995; 3:335–347.

American Gastroenterological Association. Medical position statement on obesity. *Gastroenterlogy.*2002; 123:879-881.

American Heart Association. Dietary Guidelines for Healthy Americans. Available at:http://www.aha.org.

Ascherio A, Katan MB, Zock PL, Stampfer MJ, Willett WC. Trans fatty acids and coronary heart disease. *N Engl J Med.* 1999; 340:1994–1998.

Bergen, Paul. *Medical Herbalism: A Journal for the Herbal Practitioner,* 1997.

Brand-Miller J, Wolver TM, Colagiuri S. *The Glucose Revolution: The Authoritative Guide to Glycemic Index.* New York, NY: Marlowe & Co; 1999.

Brand-Miller JC, Thomas M, Swain V, Ahmad I, Petocz P, Colagiuri S. Physiological validation of the concept of glycemic load in lean young adults. *The American Society for Nutritional sciences J. Nutur.* 2003; 133:2728-2732.

Center for Nutritional Policy and Promotion. Proposed new Daily Food Intake Patterns for Food Guide Pyramid. Available at: http://www.cnpp.usda.gov.

Chandalia M, Garg A, Lutjohann D, Von Bergmann K, Grundy SM, Brinkley LJ. Beneficial effects of high dietary fiber intake in patients with type 2 diabetes mellitus. *New England J of Med.* 2003; 42:192-1398.

Curtis B. M, O'Keefe, J. H. Understanding the Mediterranean diet. *Postgraduate medicine.* 2002; 112:2.

Delahanty LM, Halford BH. The role of diet behaviors in achieving improved glycemic control in intensively treated patients in the Diabetes Control and Complications Trial. *Diabetes Care.* 1993;16:1453–1458.

Denzer CM . The effect of resistance exercise on the thermic effect of food. *International Journal of Sport Nutrition and Exercise Metabolism* - 01-SEP-2003; 13(3): 396-402

Dueling Hunger Hormones? *Science*: 11 November 2005; 310 (5750) www.sciencemag.org/cgi/content/summary/310/5750/939.

Duggan, C. Gannon, J, Walker, W A. Protective nutrients and functional foods for the gastrointestinal tract. *Am. J. Clinical Nutrition*, May 1, 2002; 75(5): 789 - 808.

Durrant ML, Garrow JS, Royston P, Stalley SF, Sunkin S, Warwick PM. Factors influencing the composition of the weight lost by obese patients on a reducing diet. *Br J Nutr.* 1980; 44:275-285.

Ebbeling CB, Ludwig DS. Treating obesity in youth: should dietary glycemic load be a consideration? *Adv Pediatr.* 2001; 48:179-212.

Ebbeling CB, Leidig MM, Sinclair KB, Seger-Shippee LG, Feldman HA, Ludwig DS. Effects of an ad libitum low-glycemic load diet on cardiovascular disease risk factors in obese young adults. *JAMA*. 2005 Mar 9; 293(10):1189; author reply 1189-90

Ebbing CB, Leidig MM, Sinclair KB, Hangen JP, Ludwig DS. A reduced-glycemic load diet in the treatment of adolescent obesity. *Arch Pediatr Adolesc Med.*2003; 157:773-779.

Expert Panel on Detection, Evaluation, and Treatment of High Blood Cholesterol in Adults: Executive Summary of the Third Report of the National Cholesterol Education Program (NCEP) Expert Panel on Detection, Evaluation, and Treatment of High Blood Cholesterol in Adults (Adult Treatment Panel III). *JAMA.* 2001; 285:2486–2497.

Feinman RD, Fine EJ. Thermodynamics and Metabolic Advantage of Weight Loss Diets. *Metabolic Syndrome and Related Disorders* 2003; 1: 209-219.

Flatt, J. Macronutrient composition and food selection. *Obesity Research* 2001; 9:S256-S262.

Flegal KM, Carroll MD, Ogden CL, Johnson CL. Prevalence and trends in obesity among US adults. 1999-2000. *JAMA.* 2002; 288:1723-1727.

Frederick FS, Nayyar I, Parakash S, Chicano KL, Daily DA, McGory J, et al. A low-carbohydrate as compared with a low-fat diet in severe obesity. *New New England j of Med.* 2003; 348:2074-2081.

Food and Agriculture Organization (United Nations). Carbohydrates in Human Nutrition: A summary of the joint FAO/Who Expert Consultation, Rome Italy; 1997.

Garg A, Bantle JP, Henry RR, Coulston AM, Griver KA, Raatz SK, et al. Effects of varying carbohydrate content of diet in patients with non-insulin dependent diabetes mellitus. *JAMA.* 1994; 71:1421–1428.

Gertjan S. The Protein Digestibility –Corrected Amino Acid Score. *Journal of Nutrition*, 2000; 130:1865S-1867S.

Harris RB. Role of set-point theory in regulation of body weight. *FASEB J.* 1990; 4:3310-3318.

Harris JA, Benedict FG. *Biometric Studies of Basal Metabolism in Man.* Washington, DC: Carnegie Institute of Washington. 1919:279.

Hassinger W, Sauer G, Cordes U, Krause U, Beyer J, Baessler KH. The effects of equal caloric amounts of xylitol, sucrose and starch on insulin requirements and blood glucose levels in insulin-dependent diabetics. *Diabetologia.* 1981; 1:37–40.

Hensrud D. Mayo clinic on Healthy Weight. Rochester, Minn: Mayo Foundation for Medical Education and Research: 2001-2003. Available at: http://www.mayoclinic.com.

Hegsted DM, Ausman LM, Johnson JA, Dallal GE. Dietary fat and serum lipids: an evaluation of the experimental data. [Published erratum appears in *Am J Clin Nutr.*8:245, 1993]. *Am J Clin Nutr.* 1993; 57:875–883.

History of Dieting http//www.scenta.co.uk/health/features.cfm?cit_id=2568&lan_id=1&FaArea1=customWidgets.content_view_1

History diets http://shop.store.yahoo.com/carbsmart/historydiets.html

History-of-dieting http://www.thehistoryof.net/the-history-of-dieting.html

Hirsch J, Hudgins LC, Leibel RL, Rosenbaum M. Diet composition and energy balance in humans. *Am J Clin Nutr.* 1998; 67(3 suppl):551S-555S.

Institute of Medicine. Dietary reference intakes for energy, carbohydrate, fiber, fatty acids, cholesterol, protein, and amino acids. 2002. Available at: http://www.iom.edu.

International Bibliographic Information on Dietary Supplements (IBIDS) Database. http://ods.od.nih.gov/Health_Information/IBIDS.aspx

Jian V. Zhang, Pei-Gen Ren, Orna Avsian-Kretchmer, Ching-Wei Luo, Rami Rauch, Cynthia Klein, Aaron J. W. Hsueh Obestatin, a Peptide Encoded by the Ghrelin Gene, Opposes Ghrelin's Effects on Food Intake. *Science.* 11 November 2005;Vol. 310. no. 5750, pp. 996 - 999

Judd JT, Clevidence BA, Muesing RA, Wittes J, Sunkin ME, Podczasy JJ. Dietary trans fatty acids: effects on plasma lipids and lipoproteins of healthy men and women. *Am J Clin Nutr.* 1994;59:861–868.

Knowler WC, BarrettConner E, Fowler SE, Hamman RF, Lachin JM, Walker EA Nathan DM. Reduction in the incidence of type 2 diabetes with lifestyle intervention or metformin. *New England Journal of Medicine.* 2002; 346: 393-403.

Krauss RM, Eckel RH, Howard B, Appel LJ, Daniels SR, Deckelbaum RJ, et al. AHA Dietary Guidelines Revision 2000: a statement for health care professionals from the Nutrition Committee of the American Heart Association. *Circulation.* 2000;102:2284–2299.

Kris-Etherton P, Eckel RH, Howard, BV, et al. AHA science advisory. Lion diet heart study: benefits of a Mediterranean-style, National cholesterol education program/American heart association step I dietary pattern on cardiovascular disease. *Circulation.* 2001; 103 (13):1823-5.

Laura Fraser.*Losing It America's Obsession with Weight and the Industry.* New York: Penguin Press; 1998.

Levenstein ,Harvey A. *Paradox of Plenty: A Social History of Eating in Modern America* .California: University of California Press*; 2003.*

Liu S, Willett WC, Stampfer MJ, et al. A prospective study of dietary glycemic load, carbohydrate intake, and risk of coronary heart disease in US women. *Am J Clin Nutr.* 2000; 71:1455-1461.

Lichtenstein AH, Ausman LM, Jalbert SM, Schaefer EJ. Effects of different forms of dietary hydrogenated fats on serum lipoprotein cholesterol levels. [Published erratum appears in N Engl J Med341:856, 1999.] *N Engl J Med.*31999; 40:1933–1940.

Lichtenstein AH, Ausman LM, Carrasco W, Jenner JL, Ordovas JM, Schaefer EJ. Short-term consumption of a low fat diet beneficially affects plasma lipid concentrations only when accompanied by weight loss. *Arterioscler Thromb Vasc Biol.* 1994; 14:1751–1760.

Loghmani E, Rickard K, Washburne L, Vandagriff J, Fineberg N, Golden M. Glycemic response to sucrose-containing mixed meals in diets of children with insulin-dependent diabetes mellitus. *J Pediatr.* 1991; 119:531–537.

Ludwig DS, Pereira MA, Kroenke CH, Hilner JE, Van Horn L, Slattery ML, Jacobs DR Jr. Dietary fiber, weight gain, and cardiovascular disease risk factors in young adults. *JAMA*. 1999; 282(16):1529-1546.

Ludwig D. Optimal Weight for Life Program, Children's Hospital Boston], Mary V [spokeswoman for Atkins Nutritionals Inc., and coauthor of the *Atkins Diabetes Revolution]. The Lancet,* 2004; Aug. 28.

Ludwig DS. Physiological mechanisms relating to obesity, diabetes, and cardiovascular disease. *JAMA*. 2002;287:2414-2423.\

Ludwig DS. Glycemic load comes of age. *J. Nutr.* 2003; 133:2695-2696.

Luscombe ND, Clifton PM, Noakes M, Parker B, Wittert G. Effects of energy-restricted diets containing increased protein on weight loss, resting energy expenditure, and the thermic effect of feeding in type 2 diabetes. *Diabetes Care.* 2002; 25:652-657.

Madigan C, Ryan M, Owens D, Collins P, Tomkin GH. Dietary unsaturated fatty acids in type 2 diabetes. *Diabetes Care.* 2000; 23:1472–1477.

Mokdad AH, Fore ES, Bowman BA, Dietz WH, Vinicor F, Bales, VA, Marks Js. Prevalence of Obesity, Diabetes and Obesity-related Health risk factors 2001. *JAMA.* 2003;289.

National Cholesterol Education Program (NCEP) Expert Panel on Detection, Evaluation, and Treatment of High Blood Cholesterol in Adults (Adult Treatment Panel III). Third Report of the National Cholesterol Education Program (NCEP) Expert Panel on Detection, Evaluation, and Treatment of High Blood Cholesterol in Adults (Adult Treatment Panel III) final report. *Circulation.* 2002; 106:3143-3421.

National Heart, Lung and Blood Institutes. NIH Publication No. 98-4083.

National Institutes of Health; September 1998.

National Institutes of Health. Dash hypertension diet also lowers cholesterol, finds new NHLBI-funded study. National Heart Lung and Blood Institute; 2001. Available at: http://www.nih.gov.

Packer, Lester. *The Antioxidant Miracle. Canada:* Wile; 1999.

Pool, Robert. *Fat: Fighting the Obesity Epidemic*. New York: Oxford University Press; 2001, 304 pp

Pawlak DB, Kushner JA, Ludwig DS. Effects of dietary glycaemic index on adiposity, glucose homeostasis, and plasma lipids in animals. *Lancet.* 2004; 364:778-785.

Pereira MA, Swain J, Goldfine AB, Rifai N, Ludwig DS. Effects of a low-glycemic load diet on resting energy expenditure and heart disease risk factors during weight loss. *J Nutr*. 2003 Sep; 133(9):2695-6

Peristein R, Willcox J, Hines C, Milosavijevic M. Glycemic index in diabetes management. *Am Diet.*1997; 54:57-63.

Pervaz S. Resveratrol: from grapevines to mammalian biology. *The FASEB Journal*. 2003; 17:1975-1985.

Rattan S, Coxon A, Kreitzman S, Lemons A. Maintenance of weight loss with recovery of resting metabolic rate following 8 weeks of very low calorie dieting. *Int J Obes.* 1989; 13(suppl 2):189-192.

Ravnskov U. *The cholesterol myths. New Trends*, Washington, DC: Physician press; 2000.

Ravussin E, Gautier JF. Metabolic predictors of weight gain. *Int J Obes Relat Metab Disord.* 1999; 23(suppl 1):37-41.

Rickard KA, Loghmani E, Cleveland JL, Fineberg NS, Greidenberg GR. Lower glycemic response to sucrose in the diets of children with type 1 diabetes. *J Pediatr.* 1998;133:429–432.

Roberfroid, Marcel, B. Prebiotics and probiotics: are they functional foods? *American Journal of Clinical Nutrition,* Vol. 71, No. 6, 1682S-1687s, June 2000

Rolls Barbara J, Elizabeth A Bell, Victoria H Castellanos, Mosuk Chow, Christine L Pelkman, Michelle L Thorwart. Energy density but not fat content of foods affected energy intake in lean and obese women. *American Journal of Clinical Nutrition,* Vol. 69, No. 5, 863-871, May 1999

Rolls Barbara J, Roe Liane S, Jennifer S Meengs. Reductions in portion size and energy density of foods are additive and lead to sustained decreases in energy intake. *American Journal of Clinical Nutrition,* Vol. 83, No. 1, 11-17, January 2006

Salmeron J, Ascherio A, Rimm EB, Colditz GA, Spiegelman D, Jenkins DJ, et al. Dietary fiber, glycemic load, and risk of NIDDM in men. *Daibetes care.* 1997; 20:545-550.

Salmeron J, Manson JE, Stampfer MJ, Colditz GA, Wing AL, Willett WC. Dietary fiber, glycemic load, and risk of non-insulin-dependent diabetes mellitus in women. *JAMA.*1997; 277:472.

Schwartz, Hillel *Never Satisfied: A Cultural History of Diets, Fantasies, and Fat:* 1 Anchor Books, 1986.

Shick SM, Wing RR, Klem ML, McGuire MT, Hill JO, & Seagle H. Persons successful at long-term weight loss and maintenance continue to consume a low calorie, low fat diet. *Journal of the American Dietetic Association.* 1998; *98*, 408-413.

Slama G, Haardt MJ, Jean-Joseph P, Costagliola D, Goicolea I, Bornet F, et al. Sucrose taken during mixed meal has no additional hyperglycemic action over isocaloric amounts of starch in well-controlled diabetics. *Lancet* ii.1984; 122–125.

Spring B, Lieberman HR, Swope G, & Garfiel G S. Effects of carbohydrates on mood and behavior. *Nutrition Reviews Supplement*. 1986; 5. p. 52.

Steel JM, Mitchell D, Prescott RL. Comparison of the glycaemic effect of fructose, sucrose and starch-containing mid-morning snacks in insulin-dependent diabetics. *Hum Nutr Appl Nutr.* 1983; 37:3–8.

Stephenson J. Low-carb, low-fat diet gurus face off. *JAMA.* 2003; 289:1767-1773.

Stearns Peter. *Fat History, Bodies and Beauty in the Modern West :* New York University Press, 1997.

USDA. Popular weight-loss diets:U.S. Department of Agriculture White Paper. 2001;1-16.

Van Gaal LF, Rissanen AM, Scheen AJ, Ziegler O, Rössner S, for the RIO-Europe Study Group. Effects of the cannabinoid-1 receptor blocker rimonabant on weight reduction and cardiovascular risk factors in overweight patients: 1-year experience from the RIO-Europe study. *Lancet* 2005;365:1389-1397.

Westerterp KR, Wilson SA, Rolland V. Diet induced thermogenesis measured over 24h in a respiration chamber: effect of diet composition. *Int J Obes Relat Metab Disord.* 1999;23:287-292.

Willett WC, Harvard School of Public Health. *Eat, Drink, and be Healthy: The Harvard Medical School Guide to Healthy Eating.* Simon &Schuster; 2001.

Wolver TM, Jenkins DJ, Jenkins AL, Josse RG. The glycemic index: methodology and clinical implications. *Am J Clin Nutr.* 1991;54:846-854.

WEBSITES

Aerobics and Fitness Association of America
http://www.afaa.com

Alcat food allergy testing and info
www.alcat.com

Alliance for Aging Research
http://www.agingresearch.org

American Academy of Family Physicians
http://www.aafp.org

American Society of Nutrition
http://www.nutrition.org/

American College of Preventive Medicine
http://www.acpm.org

American Council on Exercise®
http://www.acefitness.org

American Counseling Association
http://www.counseling.org

American Diabetes Association
http://www.diabetes.org

American Dietetic Association
http://www.eatright.org

American Geriatrics Society
http://www.americangeriatrics.org

American Heart Association
http://www.americanheart.org

American Institute for Preventive Medicine
http://aipm.healthy.net

American Meat Institute
http://www.meatami.org

American Obesity Association
http://www.obesity.org

American Running and Fitness Association
http://www.americanrunning.org

American Society for Clinical Nutrition
http://www.faseb.org/ascn

American Society for Nutritional Sciences
http://www.faseb.org/asns

Aquatic Exercise Association
http://aeawave.com/aea.html

CDC obesity site
http://www.cdc.gov/nccdphp/dnpa/obesity/

CDC obesity trends in the USA
http://www.cdc.gov/nccdphp/dnpa/obesity/trend/maps/index.htm

Doctor Mirkin advice on nutrition and other topics
http://www.drmirkin.com

Food allergy site
http://www.woodmed.com/Food Allergy.htm

Food gateway to other sites
http://www.arborcom.com/

Harvard nutrition site – originators of GL
http://www.hsph.harvard.edu/nutritionsource/carbohydrates.html

Heart, Lung, and blood Institute
http://www.nhlbi.nih.gov/guidelines/obesity/ob_home.htm

Institute of Food Technologists
http://www.ift.org

Mayo clinic
http://www.mayoclinic.com/health/low-carb-diet/NU00279

Diabetes and food advice GI/GL list 2002
http://www.mendosa.com/gilists.htm

Mercola MD health topics
http://www.mercola.com

Metabolism web site
http://metabolism.com/

National Council on the Aging
http://www.ncoa.org

National Dairy Council
http://www.dairyinfo.com

National Food Processors Association
http://www.nfpa-food.org

National Health Council
http://www.healthanswers.com/default.asp

National Institutes of Medicine
http://www.nih.gov/

New USDA Pyramid
http://www.mypyramid.gov/

NIH/Diabetes site
http://www.niddk.nih.gov/

National Medical Association
http://www.natmed.org

National Organization for Women
http://www.now.org

National Safety Council
http://www.nsc.org

National Strength and Conditioning Association
http://www.nsca-lift.org

National Wellness Institute
http://wellnessnwi.org

Not milk- extensive articles on adverse effects of milk
www.notmilk.com

Obesity organization
http://www.obesity.org/

Obesity on line source for slides
http://www.obesityonline.org/

Office of Minority Health
http://www.omhrc.gov

Oldways Preservation Mediterranean diet pyramid
http://oldwayspt.org/

Paleolithic diet
http://paleodiet.com/

Paleolithic diet
http://www.thepaleodiet.com/

Partnership for Prevention
http://www.prevent.org

Phoenix peptide site
http://www.phoenixpeptide.com/Catalog%20Files/Ghrelin%20Section/Obestatin.html

Phytochemical and ethnobotanical database /Dr Duke
http://www.ars-grin.gov/duke/

Produce Marketing Association
http://www.pma.com

Satiation site and info to calculate caloric needs
http://www.nutritiondata.com

Surgeon general obesity site
http://www.surgeongeneral.gov/topics/obesity/

Shape Up America!
http://www.shapeup.org

Schwartz, Hillel - great reading on obesity
http://www.dimensionsmagazine.com/dimtext/Schwartz/

Tufts nutrition site
http://nutrition.tufts.edu/

University of Sidney GI/GL searchable database
http://ziag4.mmb.usyd.edu.au/mainV4a.htm

USDA food data search
http://www.nal.usda.gov/fnic/foodcomp/search/

US Gov food and nutrition center
http://www.nal.usda.gov/fnic/\

US Gov health plan
http://www.healthypeople.gov/

Weight control registry
http://www.nwcr.ws/

Veterans Administration obesity program, MOVE
http://www.move.va.gov/

Made in the USA
Monee, IL
05 November 2026

67381753R00083